AF602153

A Textbook on

Fundamentals and Applications of Nanotechnology

The Editor

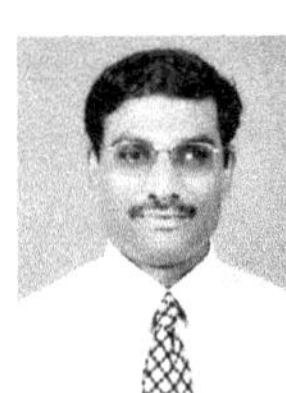

Dr. K. S. Subramanian is presently NABARD Chair Professor at the Department of Nano Science & Technology, Tamil Nadu Agricultural University Coimbatore, India. He is with the university for more than 30 years involved in teaching, research and extension activities of the university.

Dr. K. Subramanian did his Ph.D. at the University of Ottawa, Canada, utilizing one of the most prestigious Canadian Commonwealth Scholarships (1993-1998). He has got expertise in the fields of nanotechnology in agriculture and soil biology. He is the Founder Head of the Department of Nano Science & Technology and evolved the research and educational frame works in the sphere of fascinating field of nano-science and nanotechnology suiting to agricultural sciences. He is the Principal Investigator of "Enhanced Preservation of Fruits using Nanotechnology" funded by Global Affairs Canada (GAC) and International Development Research Center with a financial aid of Rs. 11.6, DST Nano Mission Projects funded by Government of India (Rs. 3 Crores) besides ICAR Nanotechnology Platform Projects. He guided more than 25 Ph.D. and Masters students' in the fields of nanotechnologies for fruit preservations, nano-fertilizers and nutrient dynamics in plant-mycorrhizal systems.

Dr. K. S. Subramanian published over 100 research papers in peer-reviewed journals and a book on Nanotechnology in Agriculture, participated as a lead speaker in various national and international conferences, visited several countries including USA, Canada, China, Taiwan, Netherlands, UAE, Sri Lanka, Tanzania, Cambodia and Ethiopia. He received more than 10 awards and distinctions to his credentials.

A Textbook on

Fundamentals and Applications of Nanotechnology

K. S. Subramanian, G. J. Janavi, S. Marimuthu
M. Kannan, K. Raja, S. Haripriya
D. Jeya Sundara Sharmila, Pon. Sathya Moorthy

2019

Daya Publishing House®

A Division of

Astral International Pvt. Ltd.

New Delhi – 110 002

ISBN 9789390384600 (PB)

Publisher's Note:

Every possible effort has been made to ensure that the information contained in this book is accurate at the time of going to press, and the publisher and author cannot accept responsibility for any errors or omissions, however caused. No responsibility for loss or damage occasioned to any person acting, or refraining from action, as a result of the material in this publication can be accepted by the editor, the publisher or the author. The Publisher is not associated with any product or vendor mentioned in the book. The contents of this work are intended to further general scientific research, understanding and discussion only. Readers should consult with a specialist where appropriate.

Every effort has been made to trace the owners of copyright material used in this book, if any. The author and the publisher will be grateful for any omission brought to their notice for acknowledgement in the future editions of the book.

Published by : **Daya Publishing House®**
A Division of
Astral International Pvt. Ltd.
– ISO 9001:2015 Certified Company –
4736/23, Ansari Road, Darya Ganj
New Delhi-110 002
Ph. 011-43549197, 23278134
E-mail: info@astralint.com
Website: www.astralint.com
Website: www.astralint.com

Digitally Printed at : **Replika Press Pvt. Ltd.**

Preface

We, authors of this book feel proud and delighted to bring out a tailor-made document to fulfill the aspirations of UG students who undertake a course on "Fundamentals and Applications of Nanotechnology". Since the course is being offered to thirteen out of fourteen degree programs and more than 2000 students take up this course every year, there is an urgent need for the synthesis of a book that covers the curriculum. Over the years, the nano-team got well equipped to deliver the course best way possible.

This book covers basic concepts and principles of nanotechnology, synthesis of nano-materials by top down (Physical) and bottom up approaches (Chemical and Biological), properties of nano-materials (physical, mechanical, optical, magnetic and thermal), characterization of nano-materials (size, stability, shape, functional group) using sophisticated equipments, application of nanotechnology in various fields (agriculture, food systems, energy, environment, health sciences) and biosafety of nano-materials (nanotoxicity and assays used for testing the nanotoxicity).

We are sure that the course content for the *"Fundamentals and Applications of Nanotechnology"* is fully covered and it is a guiding tool for the course teachers to offer the course best way possible. We take this opportunity to thank the nano-team for their contribution for the text book. We are quite sure that this book will help the teachers to effectively teach the course content regardless of their area of specialization.

Authors

Tamil Nadu Agricultural University
Coimbatore 641 003

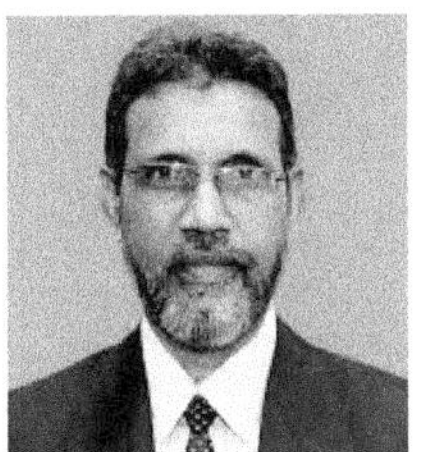

Dr. K. Ramasamy
Vice Chancellor

Foreword

Nanotechnology is a field of convergence amongst electronics, material science and biological sciences wherein atom-by-atom manipulation is performed to achieve a perfect product that is rarely possible through conventional systems. Nanotechnology has emerged as a multifarious field of science that can be applied in any disciplines. Despite its application is phenomenal in electronics, energy, environment and health sciences, we begin to scratch the surface in agricultural sciences. In India, the Tamil Nadu Agricultural University is one of the early birds in anchoring research in nano-agriculture in order to gain solutions to unresolved field problems besides transforming the conventional farming in to precision agriculture.

The paradigm shift in Indian agriculture is closely synchronized with the invigoration of agricultural education. Indeed, TNAU introduced an UG course in Nanotechnology for all degree programs with an exception of ABM for the past ten years. The course contents have been revised and revitalized to suit the needs and aspirations of agriculture graduates. A set of 12 faculty have been trained in western laboratories that helped us to build the curriculum and develop course module.

The book covers basics in nanotechnology, synthesis and characterization of nano-materials, unique properties nano-particles and applications in agriculture, food systems, health sciences, energy and environment besides biosafety. This book serves as a guiding tool for students, scholars, scientists and teachers to learn the subject and relate how best it can be integrated in their own field of specialization.

I take this opportunity to thank and congratulate the nano-team for their efforts to bring out a nice piece of reference book on *"Fundamentals and Applications of Nanotechnology"* for the UG students in any discipline in agriculture being offered by the State Agricultural Universities in the country.

Best wishes

(K. Ramasamy)

Agricultural College & Research Institute Tamil Nadu Agricultural University Coimbatore 641 003

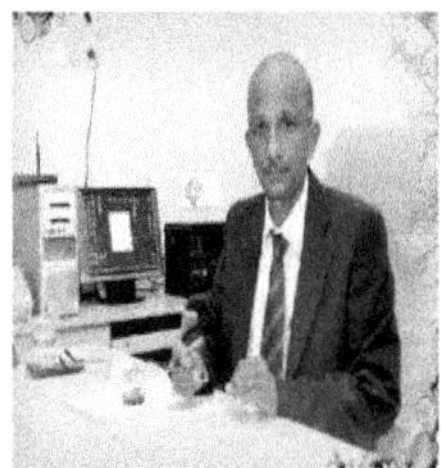

Dr. S. Mahimairaja, Ph.D.
Dean (Agriculture)

Foreword

Nanotechnology is a multi-disciplinary field involving material science, electronics and is biology, being exploited widely in energy, environment and medicine. It is a pride and deep sense of honour to express that the Tamil Nadu Agricultural University is the first State Agricultural University in India to introduce Nanotechnology which is one of the main subjects to be taught for all degree programs in agricultural sciences with an exception of B.Tech (Agri Business Management) since 2009. The University has a state-of-the-art facility to undertake teaching and research programs.

In the past eight years, the TNAU nano-team has developed and revitalized the curriculum over a period of time and the course contents have been revised in accordance with the current need and aspirations of our UG graduates. Adding further to our efforts, the Indian Council of Agricultural Research has recognized the course in the Fifth Dean's Committee.

While implementing the UG course in Nanotechnology, there is a constraint of trained faculty to teach this course in sub-campuses of TNAU and affiliated Colleges. This necessitated developing course materials in the form of a standard reference book on "Fundamentals and Applications of Nanotechnology". I am very confident that this effort will help us to deliver the course effectively across all the constituent and affiliated colleges of TNAU.

I take this opportunity to congratulate and thank the nano-team for their contribution for the text book. I am sure that this nice piece of work will help the teachers to effectively teach the course content which is fairly new to them.

Best Wishes

(S. Mahimairaja)

Contents

Contributors

Dr. G.J. Janavi Professor & Head Department of Nano Science & Technology Tamil Nadu Agricultural University Coimbatore - 641 003

Dr. K.S. Subramanian NABARD Chair Professor Department of Nano Science & Technology Tamil Nadu Agricultural University Coimbatore - 641 003

Dr. S. Marimuthu Assistant Professor (Agronomy) Department of Nano Science & Technology Tamil Nadu Agricultural University Coimbatore - 641 003

Dr. S. Haripriya Shanmugam Assistant Professor (Horticulture) Department of Nano Science & Technology Tamil Nadu Agricultural University Coimbatore - 641 003

Dr. M. Kannan Assistant Professor (Entomology) Department of Nano Science & Technology Tamil Nadu Agricultural University Coimbatore - 641 003

Dr. K. Raja Assistant Professor (Seed Science & Technology) Department of Nano Science & Technology Tamil Nadu Agricultural University Coimbatore - 641 003

Dr. M. Djanaguiraman Assistant Professor (Crop Physiology) Department of Nano Science & technology Tamil Nadu Agricultural University Coimbatore - 641 003

Dr. D. Jeya Sundara Sharmila Assistant Professor (Physics) Department of Nano Science & technology Tamil Nadu Agricultural University Coimbatore - 641 003

Dr. Pon. Sathya Moorthy Assistant Professor (Physics) Department of Nano Science & technology Tamil Nadu Agricultural University Coimbatore - 641 003

Dr. C.R. Chinnamuthu Professor (Agronomy) Department of Agronomy Agricultural College & Research Institute Tamil Nadu Agricultural University Madurai - 624 105

Dr. K. Pandian Professor Department of Inorganic Chemistry Madras University Chennai **Dr. S. K. Rajkishore**

Assistant Professor (Environ. Sciences) Agrl. College & Research Institute Kudumiyanmalai - 622104 Pudukkottai

Dr. Venkita Subbulakshmi, Chromous Biotech Private Limited, Bangalore.

1

Introduction to Nanotechnology

Dr K S Subramanian

Nanoscience and nanotechnology are the study and application of extremely small things that can be used across all the other science fields, such as chemistry, biology, physics, materials science, and engineering. The ideas and concepts behind nanoscience and nanotechnology started with a talk entitled *"There's Plenty of Room at the Bottom"* by physicist Richard Feynman at an American Physical Society meeting at the California Institute of Technology (CalTech) on December 29, 1959, long before the term nanotechnology was used. In his talk, Feynman described a process in which scientists would be able to manipulate and control individual atoms and molecules. Over a decade later, in his explorations of ultra-precision machining, Professor Norio Taniguchi coined the term nanotechnology. It wasn't until 1981, with the development of the scanning tunneling microscope that could "see" individual atoms that modern nanotechnology began.

When Neil Armstrong stepped onto the moon, he called it a small step for man and a giant leap for mankind. Nano may represent another giant leap for mankind, but with a step so small that it makes Neil Armstrong look the size of a solar system. The prefix *"nano"* means one billionth. One nanometer (abbreviated as 1 nm) is 1/1,000,000,000 of a meter. To get a sense of the nano scale, a human hair measures 80,000 nanometers across, a bacterial cell measures a few hundred nano-meters across, and the smallest features that are commonly etched on a commercial microchip as of February 2002 are around 130 nano-meters across. The smallest things seeable with the unaided human eye are 10,000 nano-meters across. Just ten hydrogen atoms and any atom in a line make up one nano-meter. It's really very small indeed. The following picture clearly illustrates the size of the nano particle. For a simple analogy, if one billion Indian populations are lined up in a one meter length, each Indian could be the size of the nano particle.

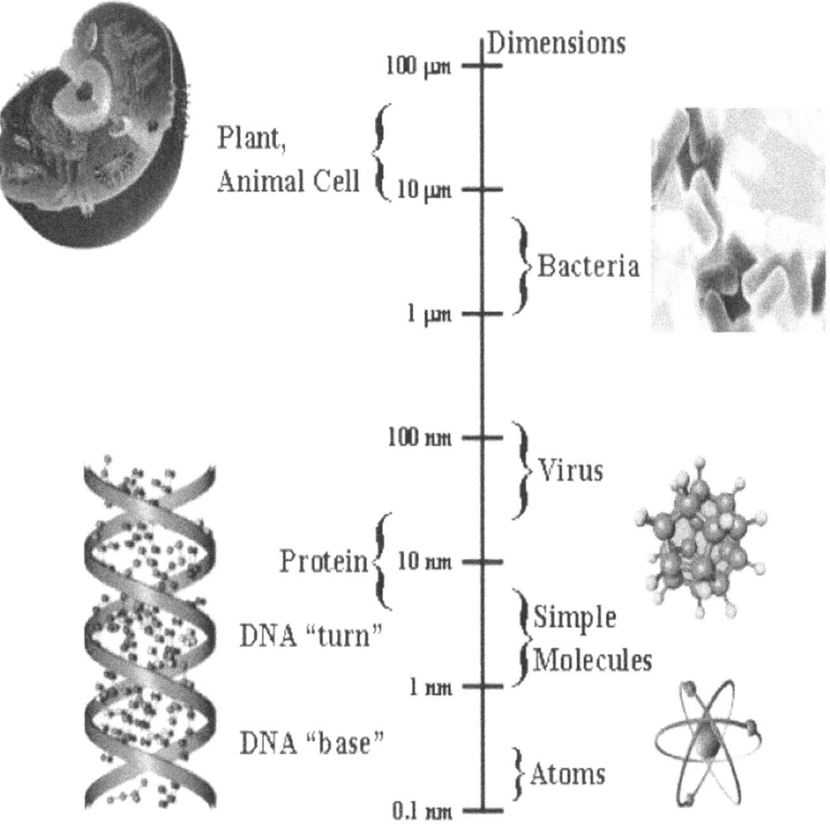

Definition

Nanoscience is, at its simplest, the study of the fundamental principles of molecules and structures with at least one dimension roughly between 1 and 100 nanometers. These structures are known, perhaps uncreative, as nanostructures. Nanotechnology is the application of these nanostructures into useful nanoscale devices. To explain that, it's important to understand that the nanoscale isn't just small, it's a special kind of small.

SI Unit Description

meter (m)	–	Approximately three feet or one yard
centimeter (cm)	–	1/100 of a meter, around half an inch
millimeter (mm)	–	1/1,000 of a meter
micrometer (µm)	–	1/1,000,000 of a meter; also called a micron,
nanometer (nm)	–	1/1,000,000,000 of a meter; the size scale of singlesmall molecules and nanotechnology

Nano Scale

Power	Prefix	Origins
10^{12}	tera	teras: monster
10^{9}	giga	gigas: giant
10^{6}	mega	megas: large
10^{3}	kilo	chilioi: thousand
10^{-3}	milli	milli: thousand
10^{-6}	micro	mikros: small
10^{-9}	nano	nanos: dwarf

History

December 29, 1959: Plenty of Room at the Bottom

A lecture of Richard Feynman delivered at the California Institute of Technology. It was titled, "There's Plenty of Room at the Bottom." Here, he proposed the "possibility of manoeuvring things atom by atom." In the book entitled "Surely your joking Mr Feynman" written in honour of him tells more about his research in the field of nanotechnology.

Mid-1970s: Nanotechnology

Idea of molecular nanotechnology, originated in the mind of Eric Drexler, when he did undergraduate in MIT. He realized that the biological 'machinery' could be adapted to build non-living products upon command.

1974: Molecular Devices

The first molecular electronic device was patented by Aviram and Seiden of IBM. Professor Norio Taniguchi of Tokyo Science University invented the term nanotechnology.

1980: Molecular Nanotechnology

K. Eric Drexler, an MIT student, writes the first paper on advanced nanotechnology.

1986: Engines of Creation

During the same time period, K. Eric Drexler publishes "Engines of Creation." Drexler presented his provocative ideas on molecular nanotechnology to a general audience.

1994: Gold Particles

Stable gold nanoparticles with molecular protection were made in solution.

"Synthesis of Thiol-Derivatised Gold Nanoparticles in a Two-Phase Liquid–Liquid System", Brust, M., M. Walker, D. Bethell, D.J. Schiffrin and R. Whyman, *J. Chem. Soc.,Chem. Commun.*, (1994), pp. 801–802.

January 1996: Assembling Molecules

Scientists at IBM succeed in moving and precisely positioning individual molecules at room temperature.

2001: Moore's Law Surpassed

In June 2001, Intel Corporation researchers announced that they had created the technology needed to produce the world's smallest and fastest silicon transistor on a mass scale. These switch on and off 5 trillion times a second.

September 2002: Molecular Electronics Breakthrough

The highest density electronically addressable memory to date has been developed. The 64-bit memory uses molecular switches. The total area is less than one square micron, giving it a bit density that is more than ten times that of current silicon memory chips.

2008: Noble prize for Physics

The Nobel Prize in Physics 2007 was awarded jointly to Albert Fert and Peter Grünberg *"for the discovery of Giant Magnetoresistance"*

2010 : Nobel prize for Graphene

Andre Geim and Kostya Novoselov were awarded the 2010 Nobel Prize in Physics "for groundbreaking experiments regarding the two-dimensional material graphene". Graphene is a form of carbon. As a material it is completely new – not only the thinnest ever but also the strongest. As a conductor of electricity it performs as well as copper. As a conductor of heat it outperforms all other known materials. It is almost completely transparent, yet so dense that not even helium, the smallest gas atom, can pass through it. Carbon, the basis of all known life on earth, has surprised us once again.

A Different Kind of Small

Imagine something we would all like to have: a cube of gold that is 3 feet on each side. Now take the imaginary cube and slice it in half along its length, width, and height to produce eight little cubes, each 18 inches (50 centimeters) on a side. The properties (excepting cash value) of each of the eight smaller cubes will be exactly the same as the properties of the big one: each will still be gold, yellow, shiny, and heavy. Each will still be a soft, electrically conductive metal with the same melting point it had before you cut it. Aside from making your gold a bit easier to carry, you won't have accomplished much at all.

Now imagine taking one of the eight 18-inch (50-centimeter) cubes and cutting it the same way. Each of the eight resulting cubes will now be 9 inches (25 centimeters) on a side and will have the same properties as the parent cube before we started cutting it. If we continue cutting the gold in this way and proceed down in size from feet to inches, from inches to centimeters, from centimeters to millimeters, and from millimeters to microns, we will still notice no change in the properties of the gold. Each time, the gold cubes will get smaller. Eventually we will not be able to see them with the naked eye and we'll start to need some fancy tools to keep cutting. Still, all the gold bricks' physical and chemical properties will be unchanged. This much is obvious from our real-world experience—at the macroscale chemical and physical properties of materials are not size dependent. It doesn't matter whether the cubes are gold, iron, lead, plastic, ice, or brass. When we reach the nanoscale, though, everything will change, including the gold's color, melting point, and chemical properties. The reason for this change has to do with the nature of the interactions among the atoms that make up the gold, interactions that are averaged out of existence in the bulk material. Nano gold doesn't act like bulk gold.

The last few steps of the cutting required to get the gold cube down to the nanoscale represent a kind of nanofabrication, or nanoscale manufacturing. Starting with a suitcase-sized chunk of gold, our successive cutting has brought it down to the nanoscale. This particular kind of nanofabrication is sometimes called top-down nanofabrication because we started with a large structure and proceeded to make it smaller. Conversely, starting with individual atoms and building up to a nanostructure is called bottom-up nanofabrication. The tiny gold nanostructures that we prepared are sometimes called quantum dots or nanodots because they are roughly dot-shaped and have diameters at the nanoscale.

The process of nanofabrication, in particular the making of gold nanodots, is not new. Much of the colour in the stained glass windows found in medieval and Victorian churches and some of the glazes found in ancient pottery depend on the fact that nanoscale properties of materials are different from macroscale properties. In particular, nanoscale gold particles can be orange, purple, red, or greenish, depending on their size. In some senses, the first nanotechnologists were actually glass workers in medieval forges rather than the bunny-suited workers in a modern semiconductor plant. Clearly the glaziers did not understand why what they did to gold produced the colours it did, but now we do.

The size-dependent properties of the nanostructures cannot be sustained when we climb again to the macroscale. We can have a macroscopic spread of gold nanodots that looks red because of the size of the individual nanodots, but the nanodots will rapidly start looking yellow again if we start pushing them back together and let them join. Fortunately, if enough of the nanodots are close to each other but not close enough to combine, we can see the red colour with the naked eye. That's how it works in the glass and glaze. If the dots are allowed to combine, however, they again look as golden as a banker's dream. To understand why this happens, nano-scientists draw on information from many disciplines. Chemists are generally concerned with molecules, and important molecules have characteristic sizes that can be measured exactly on the nanoscale: they are larger than atoms and smaller than microstructures. Physicists care about the properties of matter, and since properties of matter at the nanoscale are rapidly changing and often size-controlled, nanoscale physics is a very important contributor. Engineers are concerned with the understanding and utilization of nanoscale materials. Materials scientists and electrical, chemical, and mechanical engineers all deal with the unique properties of nanostructures and with how those special properties can be utilized in the manufacturing of entirely new materials that could provide new capabilities in medicine, industry, recreation, and the environment. The interdisciplinary nature of nanotechnology may explain why it took so long to develop. It is unusual for a field to require such diverse expertise. It also explains why most new nano research facilities are cooperative efforts among scientists and engineers from every part of the workforce.

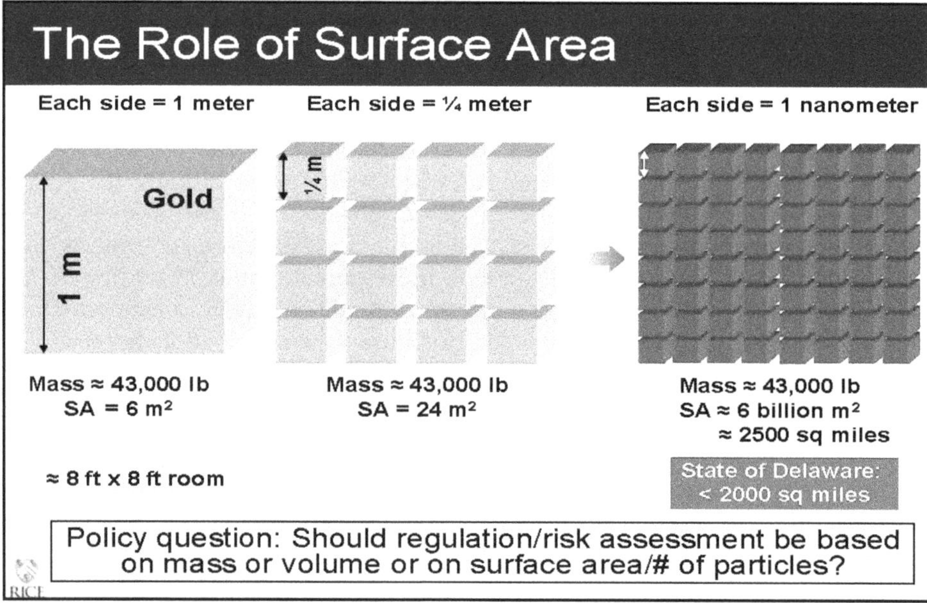

CMA (Chennai Metropolitan Area : Chennai + Thiruvallur + Kanchipuram districts) = 1170 sq. km (~500sq miles)

High Surface Mass Ratio (Unique Property)

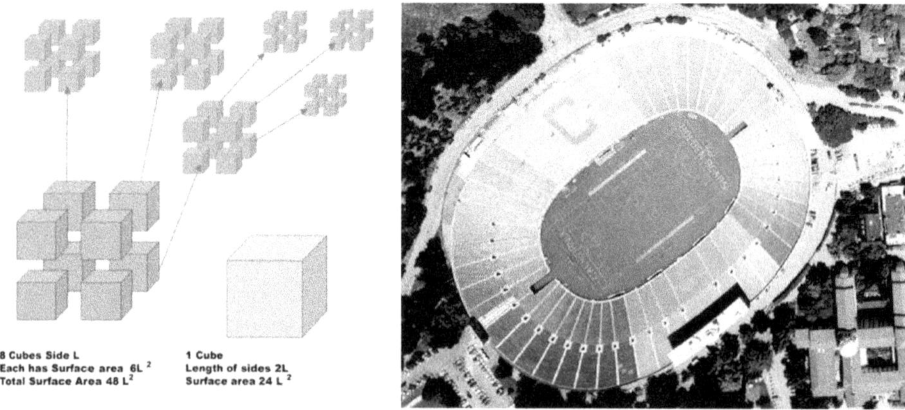

For example, 5 cm³ material divided 24 will produce 1 Nanometer cubes and spread in a single layer could cover a football field.

Some Nano Challenges

Nanoscience and nanotechnology require us to imagine, make, measure, use, and design on the nanoscale. Because the nanoscale is so small, almost unimaginably small, it is clearly difficult to do the imagining, the making, the measuring, and the using. So why bother? From the point of view of fundamental science, understanding the nanoscale is important if we want to understand how matter is constructed and how the properties of materials reflect their components, their atomic composition, their shapes, and their sizes. From the viewpoint of technology and applications, the unique properties of the nanoscale mean that nano design can produce striking results that can't be produced any other way.

Probably, the most important technological advance in the last half of the 20th century was the advent of silicon electronics. The microchip and its revolutionary applications in computing, communications, consumer electronics, and medicine were all enabled by the development of silicon technology. In 1950, television was black and white, small and limited, fuzzy and unreliable. There were fewer than ten computers in the entire world, and there were no cellular phones, digital clocks, optical fibers, or Internet. All these advances came about directly because of microchips. The reason that computers constantly get both better and cheaper and that we can afford all the gadgets, toys, and instruments that surround us has been the increasing reliability and decreasing price of silicon electronics.

Moore's Law

Gordon Moore, one of the founders of the Intel Corporation, came up with two empirical laws to describe the amazing advances in integrated circuit electronics. ***Moore's first law (usually referred to simply as Moore's law) says that the amount of space required to install a transistor on a chip shrinks by roughly half every 18 months.*** This means that the spot that could hold one transistor 15 years ago can hold 1,000 transistors today. The line gives the size of a feature on a chip and shows how it has very rapidly gotten smaller with time. Moore's first law is the good news. The bad news is Moore's second law, really a corollary to the first, which gloomily predicts that the cost of building a chip manufacturing plant (also called a fabrication line or just fab) doubles with every other chip generation, or roughly every 36 months.

Chip makers are concerned about what will happen as the fabs start churning outchips with nanoscale features. Not only will costs skyrocket beyond even the reach of current chip makers (multibillion-dollar fabs are already the norm), but since properties change with size at the nanoscale, there's no particular reason to believe that the chips will act as expected unless an entirely new design methodology is implemented. Within the next few years (according to most experts, by 2020), all the basic principles involved in making chips will need to be rethought as we shift from microchips to nanochips. For the first time since Moore stated his laws, chip design may need to undergo a revolution, not an evolution. These issues have caught the attention of big corporations and have them scrambling for their place in the nano-chip future. To ignore them would be like making vacuum tubes or vinyl records today. Aside from nanoscale electronics, one part of which, due to its focus on molecules, is often called molecular electronics, there are several other challenges that nano-scientists hope to face. To maintain the advances in society, economics, medicine, and the quality of life that have been brought to us by the electronics revolution, we need to take up the challenge of nanoscience and nanotechnology. Refining current technologies will continue to move us forward for some time, but there are barriers in the near future, and nanotechnology may provide a way to pass them. Even for those who believe that the promise is overstated, the potential is too great to ignore.

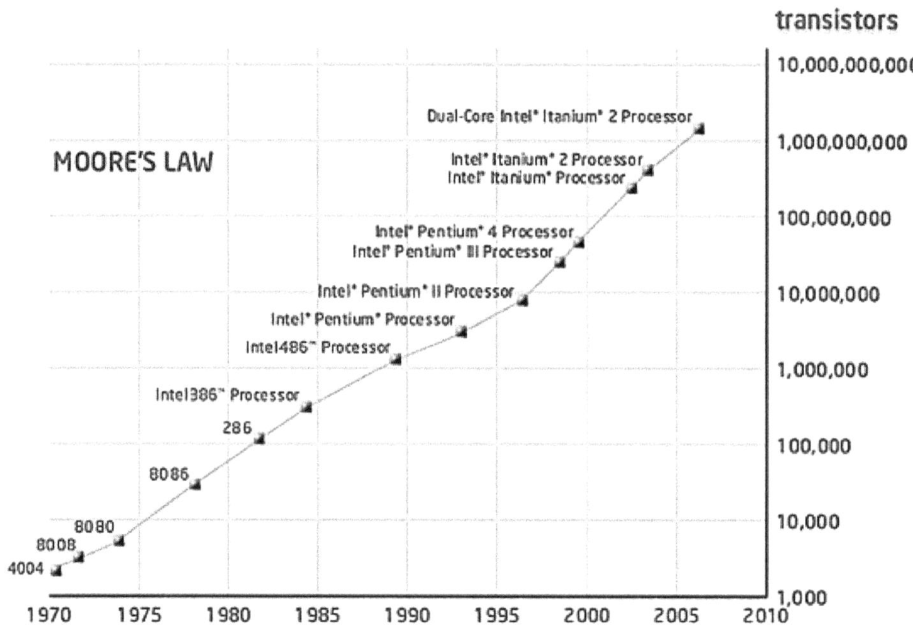

Self-assessment Questions

1. Why classic Indian arts never lose its lustre ?
2. Commonality between traditional medicine and nanotechnology ?
3. Who proposed the term "Nanotechnology"
4. What are we aiming to achieve through nanotechnology ?
5. Suggest nano-dimension of following biological specimens
   a) Viruses
   b) Haemoglobin
   c) Stomata
   d) Chlorophyll
   e) Hydrogen atom

6. State "Moore's Law"
7. Unique features of nano-particles
8. Who proposed the concept of "Plenty of Space at the Bottom"
9. How many times of division a cube should undergo to get a "nano-particle"
10. Consider that a cube has a surface area of 5 cm^3 as a macro-material and what would be the surface area when it is converted into a nano-material ?.

Fill in the blanks

1. Father of Nanotechnology is ________________

2. The Concept of "Molecular Machinery" was proposed by ________________

3. The size of the pores in leaves is ________________nm

4. The meaning of "nano" is ________________

5. Famous quote proposed by Richard Feynman is ________________

6. Gold solution was made successful in the year ________________

7. Number of nano-particles assembled across a human hair is ________________

8. Global investment in nanotechnology is ________________

Terminologies used in nanotechnology:

Ångstrom (Å): Unit of length used to measure atoms and molecules, 10^{-10} meter (m) or 0.1 nanometer (nm).

Assembler: An all-purpose device for guiding chemical reactions by positioning molecules. A programmable molecular machine, which can build any molecular structure or device from simpler chemical entities. This will be similar to an assembly machine in a factory. Originally introduced by Eric Drexler.

Atomic force microscope (AFM): A device used to get topography of a surface at atomic resolution. This is a scanning probe microscopic (SPM) device. It involves the scanning of a probe over a surface to be investigated in atomic steps.

BioNEMS: Biofunctionalized nanoelectromechanical systems. NEMS which can interact with biology.

Biopolymeroptoelectromechanical Systems (BioPOEMS): Combining optics and microelectromechanical systems which can be applied for biology.

Blue Goo: Opposite of Grey Goo. Beneficial nanobots. Grey Goo, Red Goo, Green Goo.

Bottom-up: Building larger objects starting from smaller building blocks. Starting from molecules and atoms, common approach in chemistry.

Brownian motion: Inherent motion of particles in a fluid owing to thermal agitation, named after Robert Brown (1827), its discoverer. This motion is central to many of the properties of natural systems.

Buckminsterfullerene: The spherical cage structures of carbon containing 60 atoms, resembling a football. Named after the architect Buckminster Fuller, who is famous for the geodesic domes.

Bucky balls: Short name for Buckminsterfullerene molecules.

Chemical Vapour Deposition (CVD): A technique used to prepare thin films, widely used in materials synthesis. Carbon nanotubes are largely made by this route.

Chiral: The property of an asymmetric molecule, the structure of which cannot be superimposed on its mirror image. The molecule exists in two forms called enantiomorphs, which are mirror images of each other. The solutions of these rotate the plane of polarized light in different directions, left (levo) or right (dextro), making the enantiomers levorotatory or dextrorotatory. There is also a racemic mixture, which has an equal fraction of both and therefore, will not be optically active.

Colloid: A state of matter in while particle dimension changes from that of true molecules and bulk suspensions. The dimensions vary from 1 nm to 100 nm or larger. Such solutions possess a range of properties. The particles may have charge and can be separated by electrophoresis, except at their isoelectric point (when no net charge exists). Originally, it used to refer to amorphous state, in contrast to crystalloids.

Computational nanotechnology: Computational studies of nanomaterials and structures. Almost any property of a material can be simulated.

Dendrimers: Dendrimer is a branching polymer with large molecular weight. The diversity of the branches vary depending on the generation of its growth: several of them are of nanometer dimensions. Dendrimers are used in nanoparticle synthesis.

Disassembler: An instrument able to take apart structures a few atoms at a time. See assembler.

DNA chip: A chip built to identify mutations or alterations in the DNA code.

Dry nanotechnology: Fabrication of nanostructures without biology or wet chemistry. A carbon nanotube based technology will be dry as against a technology with DNA which will be 'wet'. See wet nanotechnology. These two terms were originally introduced by Prof. R.E. Smalley.

Femtotechnology: Manipulating materials on the scale of elementary particles (leptons, hadrons, and quarks). A technology after picotechnology, which is below the length scale of nanotechnology. Also used as Femtotech.

Fullerenes: Fullerenes are a molecular form of pure carbon discovered in 1985 and rewarded with a Nobel Prize for the discoverers (Kroto, Smalley and Curl) in 1996. They are cage-like structures of carbon atoms, the most abundant form produced is buckminsterfullerene (C60), with 60 carbon atoms arranged in a spherical structure. There are larger fullerenes containing from 70 to 500 carbon atoms. Various other forms of fulleneres are now known, even with other elements.

Functionalized / functionalization: The attachment of a chemically active moieties to an inert molecule/ entity.

Gray Goo or Grey Goo: Destructive nanobots. opposite of Blue Goo. Several other Goo's have been proposed.

Langmuir-Blodgett (LB) method: A technique used to make ultrathin films, first a Langmuir film is made (at air-liquid interface) which is then compressed and transferred to a substrate.

MEMS: Microelectromechanical systems: generic term to describe micron scale electrical/mechanical devices.

Molecular integrated microsystems (MIMS): Microsystems in which functions found in biological and nanoscale systems are integrated with materials.

Molecular mechanics: A method by which the molecular potential energy function is computed to understand and predict various properties of the system.

Moore's law: Coined by Gordon Moore originally in 1965, Chairman and Chief Executive of Intel. The of number transistors packed into an integrated circuit had doubled every year since the technology's inception four years earlier. In 1975, the time period was revised to every two years. People use a time scale of 18 months, which is obeyed approximately all through the semiconductor revolution.

Nano-assembler: A nanoscale device which combines individual molecules into the structures required.

Nanobiotechnology: Application of nanotechnology to learn biological systems and use of this knowledge for devices and methods.

Nanobot: Nanorobot or Nanomachine.

Nanobubbles: Nanosized bubbles with or without molecules or objects. We have a chapter on such objects in this volume.

Nanochips: Next generation chips with higher storage density.

Nanoclusters: Aggregates of atoms, molecules or clusters in the nanoscale.

Nanocrystals: Crystals of elements or compounds in the nanoscale, with which they manifest properties different from their bulk counterparts. The crystal structure may be the same or different from their bulk analogues.

Nanofabrication: Fabrication of materials and devices using assemblers starting from molecules, same as nanoscale engineering.

Nanofilters: Objects used for selective filtration of molecules depending on their sizes.

Nanofluidics: The study of manipulation of nanoscale quantities of fluids.

Nanoimprinting: Also called soft lithography. A technique developed by Whitesides and co-workers using mould based printing, the moulds have nanoscale features. The creations of features sometimes utilize self assembled monolayers (SAMs).

Nanoindentation: Force exerted by a diamond indenter is measured as it makes an indent of nanometer dimensions in a material. The stiffness and hardness of the material are extracted. Mechanical properties of the material are understood from such studies.

Nanolithography: Nanoscale writing.

Nanomachine: A molecular machine made to perform mechanical functions.

Nanomachining: Machining of matter by modifying materials in the nanoscale.

Nanomanipulator: A virtual reality device connected to a scanning probe microscope, allowing manipulation of atoms. Here individual molecules, DNA and atomic objects can be manipulated. Nanomanipulation refers to the process.

Nanomanufacturing: Molecular manufacturing.

Nanomaterials: Materials in which one of the dimensions of the constituent objects is under 100 nm.

Nanometer (nm): 10^{-9}m.

Nanooptics: Investigation of light-matter interaction at the nanoscale.

Nanopens and Nanopencils: Objects used in dip pen lithography allowing drawing of objects for nanoelectronics.

Nanopharmaceuticals: Use of nanoscale objects for the use of delivery, transport, uptake and delivery of pharmaceuticals.

Nanopipettes: Objects similar to pipettes with which controlled delivery of chemicals, reagents and light at nanometer scale areas. An area of research used intensely in biology for manipulating living organisms.

Nanopores: Channels with dimension as small as single molecules or DNA which can be used for molecular separation. This pores can be in membranes, ceramic objects such as zeolites. This kind of objects can simplify biomolecular separation.

Nanoprobe: Nanoscale devices used to understand the properties of materials and systems.

Nanoreplicators: A nanobot capable of replication.**Nanorods:** Objects with diameter in the nanodimension, length can be from nanometers to microns. Several nanorods are known, with metals and semiconductors.

Nanoropes: Nano objects such as particles, rods and tubes connected to form a rope.

Nanoscale: The dimension of 1-100 nm.

Nanosensor: Sensor for chemical or physical properties made with nanomaterials.

Nanoshells: Shells with wall thickness or dimension in the nanoscale. Nanoshells of metals, semiconductors, insulators and polymers are known. We have a chapter on this in the volume. Also used as nanobubbles.

Nanosystem: An assemblage of nanoscale components designed for a specific function.

Nanotube: A cylindrical tube of carbon with diameter in the range of nanometers and length of the order of microns, discovered by Sumio Iijima, 1991.

Nanowires: Similar to nanorods, but of longer length than rods.

NEMS: Nanoelectromechanical systems: Nanoscale electrical/mechanical devices.

Pico technology: Next smaller step after Nanotechnology.

Quantum: A discrete quantity of electromagnetic radiation or amount of energy associated with a process.

Quantum dots: Nanocrystals or nanoparticles. Refer to confined electrons. Electrons in them occupy discrete states as in the case of atoms and therefore, quantum dots are referred to as artificial atoms.

Red Goo: Refers to designed nanotechnological objects for destruction, similar to grey goo, which is accidentally created.

Self-assembly: Molecular organization without external stimulus.

Self-repair: Ability to heal itself without external influence.

Self-replication: An ability of an assembler to replicate itself to a definite amount within a fixed period.

SEM: Scanning electron microscopy, imaging technique in which a focused beam of electrons is used to scan the sample and the generated secondary electrons and ions as well as deflected primary electrons are used to image the sample.

Smart materials: Products with ability to respond to the environment, such as shape transformation.

Spintronics: Electronic devices exploiting the spin of electrons, in addition to charge.

SPM: Scanning probe microscope (SPM), including AFMs and STMs, in which effect of interaction of a sharp probe with the sample is measured to infer atomic structure of the material.

STM: Scanning tunneling microscopy, also Scanning thermal microscopy, Imaging technqie using local temperature variations of the sample.

Superlattices: Materials which exhibit double periodicity. A nanoparticle can be crystallized into a superlattice in which there will be a periodicity within the nanoparticle (gold lattice for example) and a periodicity of the particles themselves. Such superlattices are known in conventional materials also, in addition to multilayered films.

Top-down approach: Making nanosystems, materials and devices starting from bulk materials.

Tunneling: A truly quantum mechanical effect due to the wave nature of matter by which a particle can cross over a barrier if its wave function has a finite probability of existence.

UHV: Ultra high vacuum, a requirement of most of the high quality scientific instrumentation, considered as vacuum better than 10^{-8} torr.

Van der Waals force: Weak intermolecular attractive forces.

Wet nanotechnology: Bionanotechnology, where nanosystems function in the presence of water. The nanomaterials are membranes, enzymes and such biological entities. All life is based on such technologies.

2

Classification of Nanomaterials based on Origin and Dimension, brief Introduction to Quantum Dots, Buckyball, Carbon Nanotube

Dr. D. Jeya Sundara Sharmila

Classification of Nanomaterials based on Dimension

Nanostructured materials derive their special properties from having one or more dimensions made small (<100nm) compared to a length scale critical to the physics of the process. Nanomaterials can be classified according to the following categories *i.e.,* **Size:** Any one dimension is < 100 nm across; Origin: Natural, Incidental or Engineered; **Form:** Amorphous, crystalline, polymeric or composites; **Shapes:** Spheres, tubes, rods, cones and fibers *etc;* Non-metal (e.g., carbon), metallic (e.g., Au, Ag), semiconductor (e.g., Cd-Se), or a combination. Their physical properties are related to their size and chemical compositions.

Classification based on the number of dimensions, which are not confined to the nanoscale range (<100 nm) are: zero-dimensional (0-D), one-dimensional (1-D), two-dimensional (2-D), and three-dimensional (3-D) (Fig. 1).

Zero-dimensional Nanomaterials

Materials wherein all the dimensions are measured within the nanoscale i.e., less than 100nm. (no dimensions, or 0-D, are larger than 100 nm). The most common representation of zero-dimensional nanomaterials are nanoparticles.

One-dimensional Nanomaterials

Only one dimension is outside the nanoscale. This leads to needle like-shaped nanomaterials. 1-D materials include nanotubes, nanorods and nanowires.

Two-dimensional Nanomaterials

Two of the dimensions are not confined to the nanoscale. 2-D nanomaterials exhibit plate-like shapes. Two-dimensional nanomaterials include nanofilms, nanolayers, and nanocoatings.

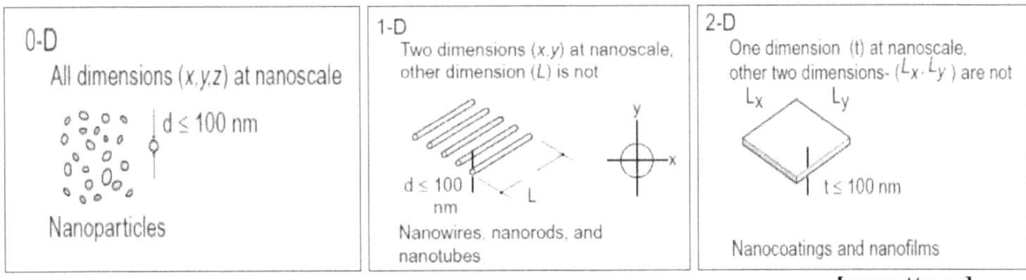

[www.ttu.ee]

Figl

Three-dimensional Materials

Bulk materials are materials that are not confined to the nanoscale in any dimension. These materials are thus characterized by having three arbitrarily dimensions above 100 nm. Materials possess a nanocrystalline structure or involve the presence of features at the nanoscale. In terms of nanocrystalline structure, bulk nanomaterials can be composed of a multiple arrangement of nanosize crystals, most typically in different orientations (Fig. 2). With respect to the presence of features at the nanoscale, 3-D nanomaterials can contain dispersions of nanoparticles, bundles of nanowires, and nanotubes as well as multi-nanolayers.

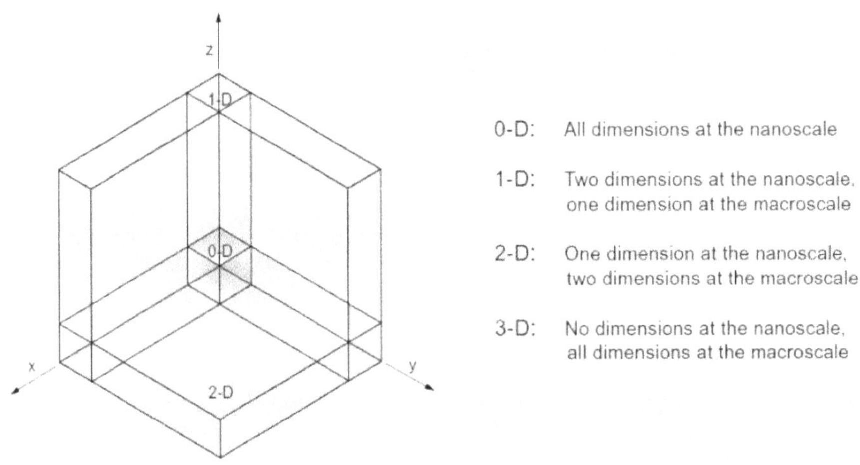

[www.ttu.ee]

Fig. 2

Nanomaterials can be amorphous or crystalline, single crystalline or polycrystalline, composed of single or multi-chemical elements. They can exhibit various shapes and forms, exist in individually or incorporated in a matrix, metallic, ceramic, or polymeric.

Origin based Classification

Natural originated nanoparticles: Sea spray, Natural mineral composites, Volcanic ash, Viruses, Fine sand and dust.

Manmade anthropogenic incidental nanoparticles are produced as a result of by-product of process such as by product of combustion, industrial manufacturing, and other human activities- cooking smoke, diesel exhaust, welding fumes, industrial effluents, large-scale mining coal fly ash, industrial effluents, sandblasting. They are poorly controlled in size and shape and jumble of different elements.

An engineered nanomaterial is any intentionally produced material that has a size in 1, 2, or 3-dimensions of typically between 1-100 nm. They are very precisely controlled in sizes, shapes, and compositions. Ex.: Metal NPs, Quantum dots, Buckyballs / Fullerene, Carbon Nanotubes, Sunscreen pigments, nano capsules.

Nanoparticle classifications based on its Composition: Metals, Metal oxides, Carbonaceous: Fullerenes and Carbon Nanotubes, Semiconductors (Quantum dots), Polymers (dendrimers), Ceramics, Composites.

Brief Introduction to Quantum Dots, Buckyball, Carbon Nanotube

Quantum Dots (QD)

Discovered in1980 by Alexei Ekimovin & Louis Brusin and the term "Quantum Dot" was coined by Marl Reed. The size of Quantum Dots range from 2 to 10 nanometers in diameter (about the width of 50 atoms). They emit photons (light) under excitation, (when stimulated by an external source such as ultraviolet (UV) light) which are visible to the human eye as light. The wave length of the photon emission from Quantum Dot depends on the size of the quantum dots. The size of the quantum dots can be precisely controlled during synthesis. The ability to precisely control the size of a quantum dot enables the manufacturer to determine the wavelength of the emission, which in turn determines the colour of light the human eye perceives. Quantum dots can therefore be "tuned" during production to emit any colour of light desired (Fig. 3).

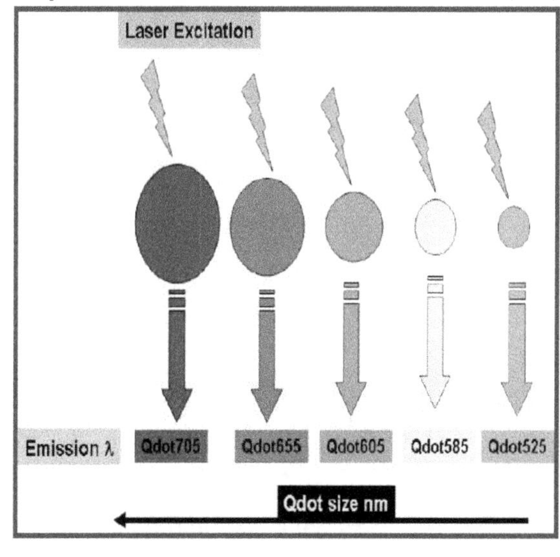

Fig. 3 [www.icms.qmul.ac]

The smaller the dot, the closer it is to the blue end of the spectrum, and the larger the dot, the closer to the red end. Dots can even be tuned beyond visible light, into the infra-red or into the ultra-violet.

Potential Applications of QD

Drug discovery, Diagnostics, Biological reagents, Genetic analysis, Solid-state lighting, Sensors, Display screens, Cosmetics and Solar cells

Buckyballs

Buckyball (buckminster fullerene) is an allotrope of carbon (C_{60}). They were discovered as an unexpected surprise during laser spectroscopy experiments conducted by Robert Curl, Harold Kroto and Richard Smalley at Rice University in September 1985. Allotropes are different structural forms of the same element (Fig. 4). The atoms of the element are bonded together in a different manner and exhibit quite different physical and chemical behaviours. Elements such as carbon, oxygen, phosphorus, tin and sulfur, display allotropy.

Allotropes of carbon have different covalent bonding arrangements

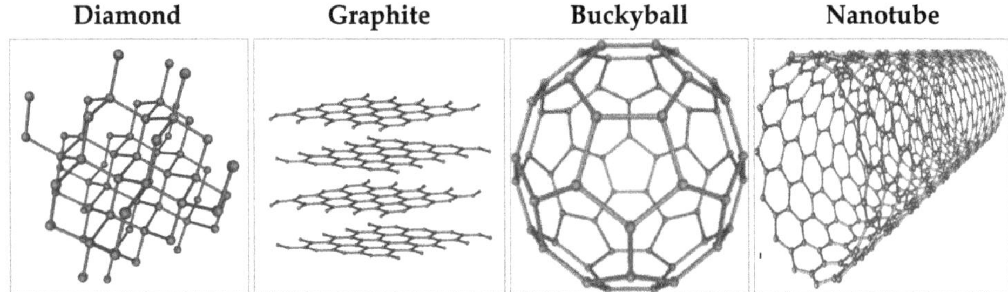

Fig. 4

Fullerenes are named after architect Richard Buckminster Fuller, due to their similarity to his geodesic dome design (a type of structure shaped like a piece of a sphere or a ball) and are often referred to as "buckyballs" (Fig. 5).

Structure of C60

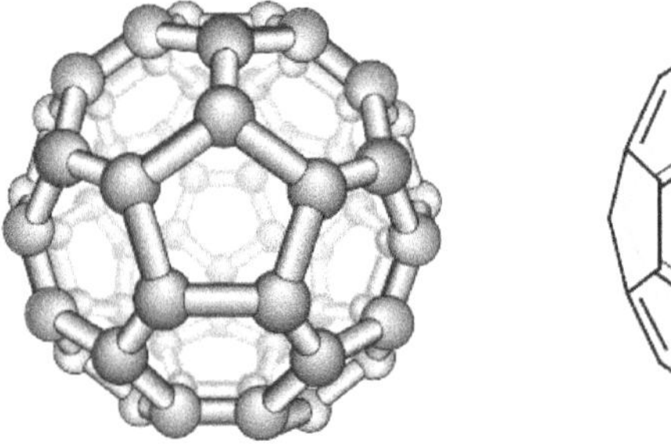
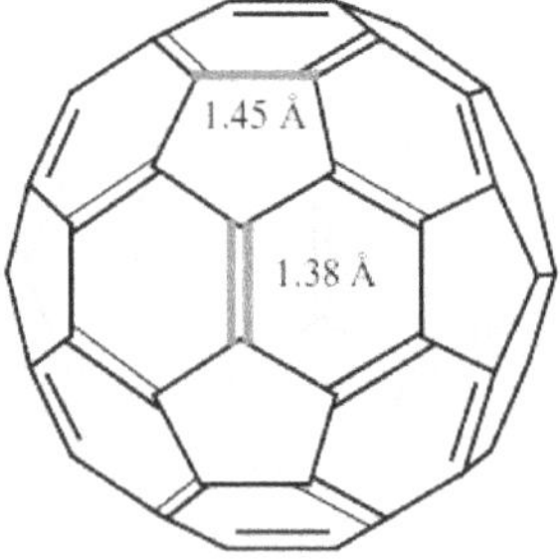

20 hexagonal faces + 12 pentagonal faces

Fig. 5

Carbon Nanotube (CNT)

Discovered in 1991 by the Japanese electron microscopist Sumio Iijima. Originally called "buckytubes" but now are called as carbon nanotubes or CNT for short. Carbon nanotubes are in the structural family of fullerene. Carbon nanotubes / buckytubes are allotropes of carbon with a cylindrical nanostructure. They are molecules composed entirely of carbon atoms. Length from several hundred nm to μm, diameter of 0.4-2 nm (SWNT) and 2 -100nm (MWNT). CNT can be described as a sheet of graphite (graphene) rolled into a cylinder (Fig. 6). They are constructed from hexagonal rings of carbon and can have one layer or multiple layers.

Types of Carbon Nanotubes

Single walled CNT differs based on symmetry into armchair, zig-zag and chiral(helical). The carbon nanotubes can be thought of as graphene planes 'rolled up' in a cylinder. Depending on how the grapheme plane is 'cut' and rolled up, three types of carbon nanotubesare obtained.

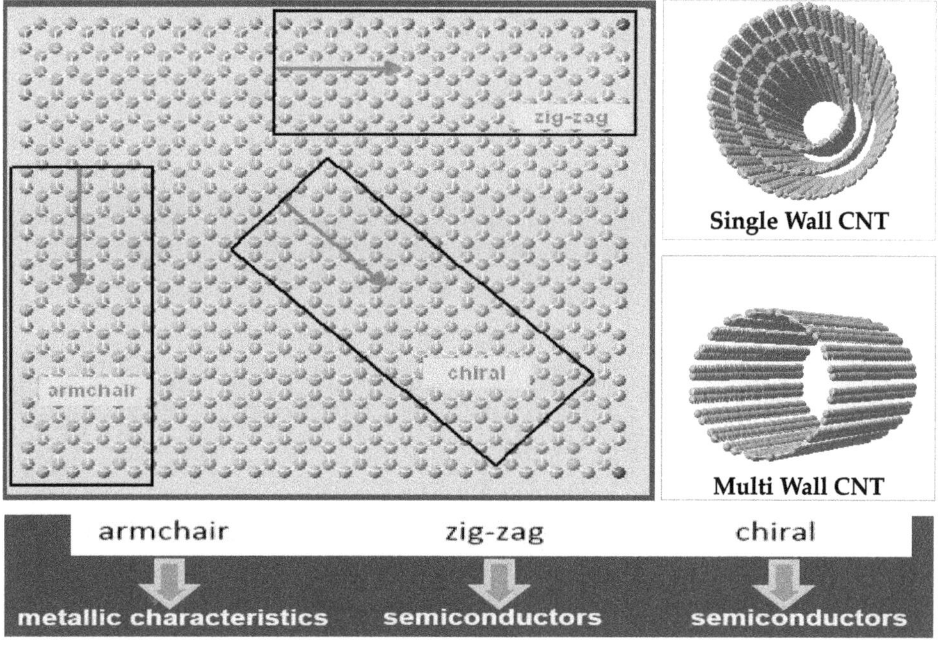

Fig. 6 **[academic.pgcc.edu]**

Self-assessment Questions

1. Single walled CNT differs based on symmetry into _____ (Armchair, Zig-Zag and Chiral).
2. Nanomaterials wherein all the dimensions are measured within the 100 nm are _______ (0 Dimensional)

3. QDs were discovered by ________________ (Alexei Ekimovin & Louis Brusin)
4. ________ are not confined to the nanomaterial range in any dimension (BulK).
5. ________________are different structural forms of the same element (Allotropes).
6. Fullerenes are named after the architect ____________ (Richard Buckminster Fuller)
7. CNT was discovered in 1991 by ________ (Sumio Iijima)

3

Unique Properties of Nanomaterials – Physical, Chemical and Optical Properties

Dr. Jeya Sundara Sharmila

Nanomaterials are (Nano = 10^{-9}m) one billionth in size and with dimensions and tolerances in the range of 100 nm to 0.1 nm. At the nanometer scale, the various physical and chemical properties of materials become size-dependent.

1. Physical properties – Mechanical hardness, Fracture strength, Density etc
2. Chemical properties – Thermal Melting temperature, Lattice constant
3. Optical properties – absorption and scattering of light
4. Electrical properties – tunneling current
5. Magnetic properties – Superparamagnetic effect

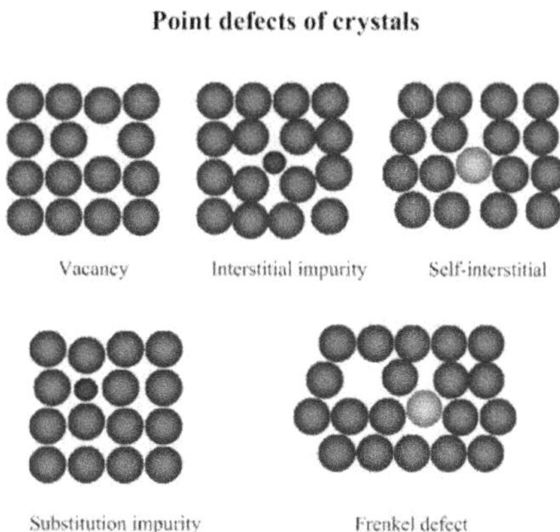

Fig. 3.1

Physical Properties of Nanomaterials

The basic properties of nanomaterials are the results of the physics and chemistry of solids depend on the microstructure. Microstructure in term classified into, (a) chemical composition- the arrangement of the atoms (the atomic structure) & (b) the size of a solid in one, two or three dimensions. Physical (Mechanical) parameters influencing structure are atomic defects, dislocations and strains, grain boundaries and interfaces, porosity, connectivity and percolation, short range order etc. **Defects** are usually absent in either metallic or ceramic clusters of nanoparticles because dislocations are basically unstable or mobile **(Fig. 1).** When these clusters are assembled under uniaxial pressure into a pellet, a fully consolidated nanophase material looks very much like a normal, dense polycrystalline aggregate, but at a far smaller scale. A **grain** is a single crystal within a bulk/thin films form. **Plasticity** is defined as the property of material remain deformed after the force is removed. **Creep** is the tendency of a solid material to move slowly or deform permanently under the influence of mechanical stresses. Crystals contain internal interfacial defects, known as **grain boundaries**, where the lattice orientation changes

Hall-Pelch Effects

The Hall-Petch relation (law) gives a quantitative description of an **increase in the yield stress of a polycrystalline material as its grain size decreases.** This relationship is based on dislocation mechanisms of plastic deformation i.e., grain boundaries hinder the movement of dislocations. The variation in strength can be described by a power-law relationship **(Fig. 2)**

$$\sigma_y = \sigma_0 + k_d/d^{1/2}$$

Where

σ_y - yield stress,

K_d - Strengthening coefficient,

d - the average grain diameter

σ_0 - materials constant for the starting stress for dislocation movement (or the resistance of the lattice to dislocation motion)

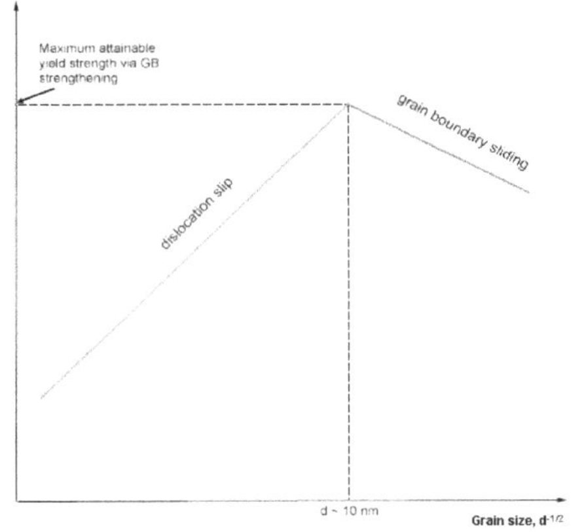

Fig. 2

Hall-Petch Strengthening Limit

Hall-Petch Strengthening is limited by the size of dislocations. Once the grain size reaches about 10 nm, grain boundaries start to slide. At the smallest grain sizes all deformation is accommodated in the grain boundaries and grain boundary sliding, a process based on mechanical and thermally activated single atomic jumps, dominates the contribution to deformation. At large grain sizes, a combination of sliding and intra-grain dislocation activity is observed. At the smallest grain sizes all the deformation is accommodated in the grain boundaries. At larger grain sizes lattice dislocation activity is observed. At smaller grains sizes a gradual reduction of the modulus is observed. Dislocation is a line defect within a crystal which arises during crystal growth or as a results of mechanical deformation of a crystal **(Fig. 3).**

Diffusion Creep

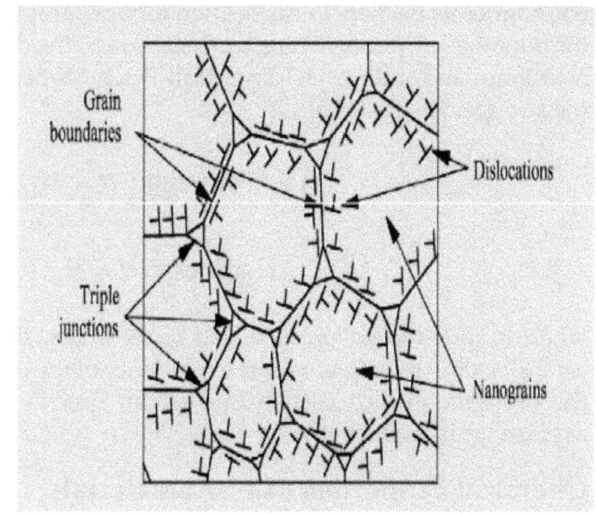

Fig. 3

Diffusion creep is caused by the migration of crystalline defects through the lattice of a crystal such that when a crystal is subjected to a greater degree of compression in one direction relative to another, defects migrate to the crystal faces along the direction of compression, causing a net mass transfer that shortens the crystal in the direction of maximum compression. Diffusion creep results in plastic deformation rather than brittle failure of the material. Diffusion creep is more sensitive to temperature than other deformation mechanisms. It usually takes place at high homologous temperatures (*i.e.* within about a tenth of its absolute melting temperature). The migration of defects is in part due to vacancies, whose migration is equal to a net mass transport in the opposite direction.

Stress – Strain Curve

Stress is force per unit area causing the deformation. Strain is a measure amount of deformation. The elastic modulus is the constant of proportionality between stress and strain (Fig. 3.4a). Hardness is a measure of how resistant solid matter is to various kinds of permanent shape change when a compressive force is applied **(Fig. 4 b).**

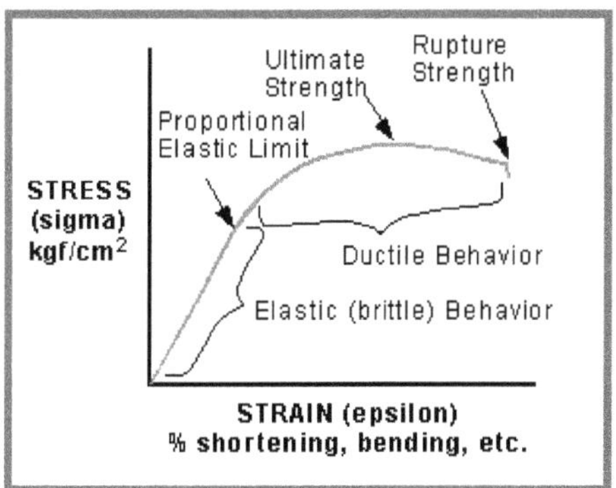

Fig. 4 a

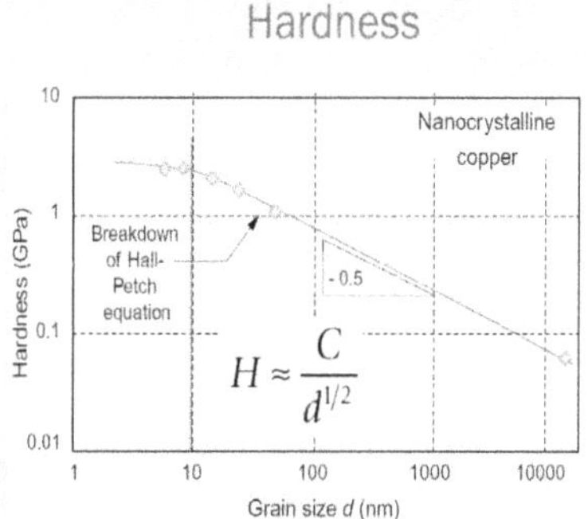

Fig. 4 b

Fracture toughness is a property which describes the ability of a material containing a crack to resist fracture, and is one of the most important properties of any material for many design applications. The Hall-Petch model treats grain boundaries as barriers to dislocation motion, and thus dislocations pile up against the boundary. Upon reaching a critical stress, the dislocations will cross over to the next grain and induce yielding. Hall Petch Model says the smaller the grain size the stronger the material.

$$\text{Yield strength: } \sigma_{TS} = \sigma_O + \frac{K_{TS}}{\sqrt{d}}$$

$$\text{Hardness: } H = H_O + \frac{K_H}{\sqrt{d}}$$

where σ_{TS} is the yield stress, σ_o and H_0 are materials constant for the starting stress for dislocation movement (or the resistance of the lattice to dislocation motion), K is the strengthening coefficient (a constant specific to each material), and *d* is the average grain diameter.

Chemical Properties of Nanomaterials

Reason for the material size < 100 nm having a lower melting point (the difference can be as large as 1000 deg C) and reduced lattice constant is the dramatic changes in surface energy to volume energy ratio. What is easier to get off? Surface atom or Volume atom **(Fig. 5)**

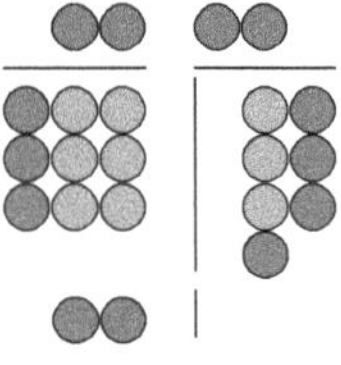

Fig. 5

Melting Points and Lattice Constants

Atoms or molecules on a solid surface possess fewer nearest neighbors or coordination numbers, and thus have dangling or unsatisfied bonds exposed to the surface. Because of the dangling bonds on the surface, surface atoms or molecules are under an inwardly directed force and the bond distance between the surface atoms or molecules and the subsurface atoms or molecules, is smaller than that between interior atoms or molecules. When solid particles are very small, such a decrease in bond length between the surface atoms and interior atoms becomes significant and the lattice constants of the entire solid particles show an appreciable reduction.

Surface Energy

The extra energy possessed by the surface atoms is described as surface energy, surface free energy or surface tension. Surface energy, by definition, is the energy required to create a unit area of "new" surface. Concepts of thermodynamics are used to calculate the surface energy of a material.

$$\gamma = \left(\frac{\partial GibbsfreeEnergy}{\partial Area} \right)_{@constpressure, temp, number}$$

Gibbs free energy (G) is defined as the energy portion of a thermodynamic system available to do work.

$\Delta G = \Delta H - T\,\Delta S$; H is the enthalpy, T is the temperature and S is the entropy (disorder).

If one keep cutting to increase the overall surface free energy and Gibbs Free Energy by increasing the number of free bonds (H internal energy) **(Fig. 6)**

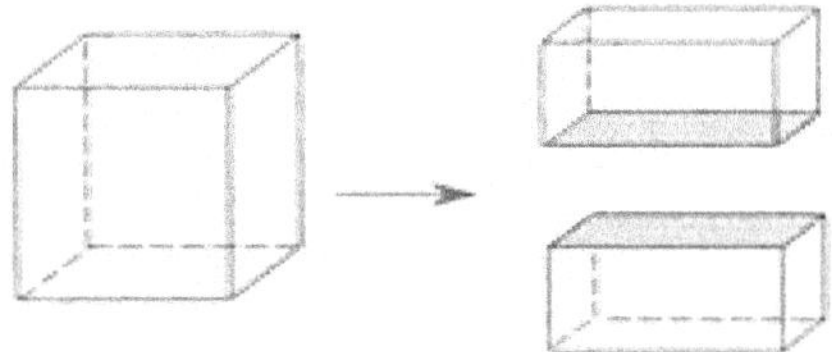

Fig. 6

Surface energy is expressed for most materials a first order estimate is given by:

$$\gamma = 1/2 n_b \varepsilon$$

bondstrength in the bulk (close enough assumption)

number of broken bonds per unit area on the new surface

Magnetic Properties of Nanomaterials

Magnetic properties of nanostructured materials are distinctly different from that of bulk materials. Ferromagnetism disappears and transfers to superparamagnetism **(Fig. 7)** in the nanometer scale due to the huge surface energy.

Table 1: Types of Magnetism (H is applied field and M is magnetization)

Magnetism	Susceptibility	Critical temperature	Atomic behavior	Magnetic behavior
Diamagnetism	Small & negative	None		M H
Paramagnetism	Small & positive	None		M H
Ferromagnetism	Large & positive	Curie		M H
Anti-ferromagnetism	Small & positive	Neel		M H
Ferrimagnetism	Large & positive	Curie		M H
Super-paramgnetism	Large & positive	Curie		M H

Paramagnet, Ferromagnet & Superparamagnets

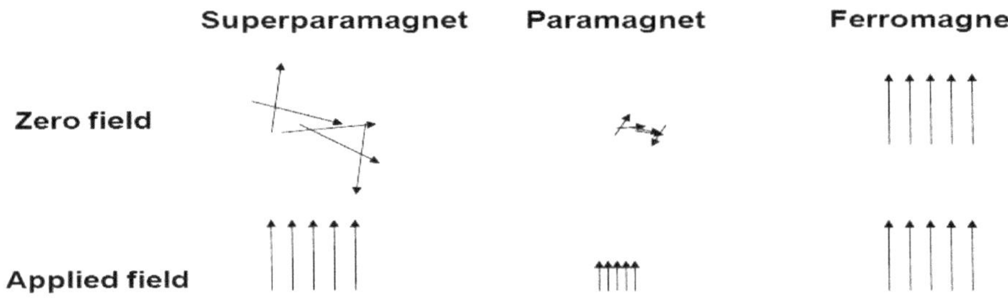

Fig. 7

	Superparamagnet	Paramagnet	Ferromagnet
at Zero Magnetic Field	Domain moments that would couple as in Ferromagnet do not do so because of small size—boundary effect.	Domain moments align randomly—no net moment.	Domain moments coupled (below Curie temp.) to produce strong, permanent moment.
at Magnetic Field Applied	Domains "find" each other and now it generates a moment comparable to Ferromagnet.	Net moment appears; the applied magnetic field helps the domains "find" each other to become coupled.	Even higher magnetic moment.

Superparamagnets are considered as a small ferromagnet, because of its small size, the magnetic moment wanders. When given an order to align (when a magnetic field is imposed) it aligns with the same enthusiasm that a ferromagnet has, which exceeds that of the paramagnet. Like the paramagnet, the superparamagnets return to zero magnetization when the field is removed **(Fig. 8 a & b).**

Application of Super-paramagnetic Nanoparticles

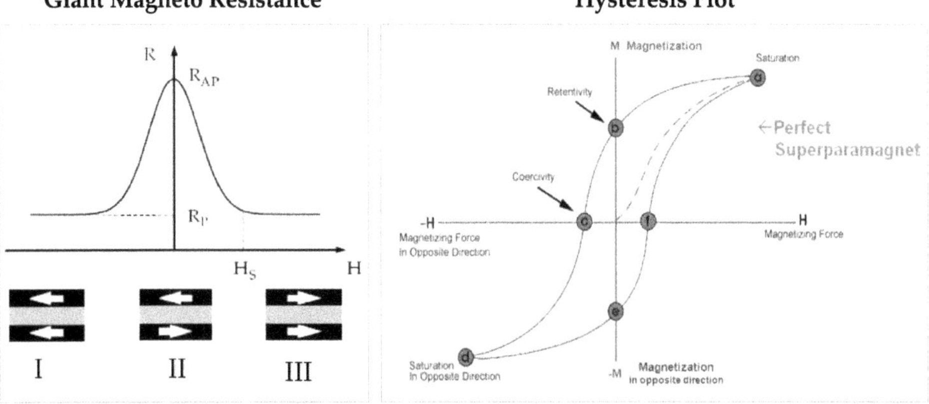

Fig. 8 a

Fig. 8 b

[uab.edu]

Nano particles can have very high magnetic susceptibility with permanent magnetic dipole. Small clusters consisting of a single ferromagnetic domain follow the applied field freely (super-paramagnetism). The magnetic susceptibility of superparamagnetic particles is orders of magnitude larger than bulk paramagnetic materials. Giant magnetoresistance occurs when the magnetic layers above and below the conductor are magnetized in opposite direction. Electron scattering in magnetic media is strongly dependent on spin polarization. When magnetic layers are locally magnetized, only one spin polarization is scattered (I, III). For antiparallel magnetic layers both spin polarizations are scattered, giving rise to super-resistance (II) **(Fig. 8a).** Magnetic hard drives are based on a nanostructured device, called giant magnetoresistance sensor (Albert Fert, Peter Grünbers Nobel Prize in Physics 2007). The magnetization on the surface of the disk can be read out as fluctuations in the resistance of the conducting layer.

Magnetic Nanowires

Example: Cobalt nanowires on Si substrate (Fig. 3.9), Cobalt, gold, copper and cobalt-copper nanowire arrays Important for storage device applications

Electrochemical deposition is the fabrication technique <20 nm diameter nanowire arrays can be fabricated by electrochemical deposition.

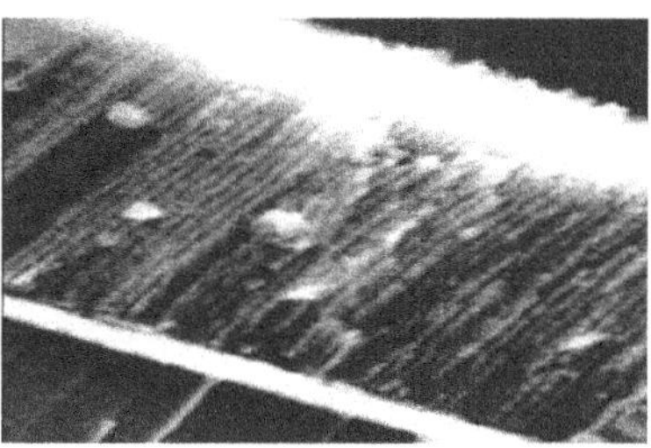

Fig. 9.
(Umass Amherst, 2000)

Electrical Properties of Nanomaterials

Nanocrystalline particles represent a state of matter in the transition region between bulk solid and single molecule. As a consequence, their physical and chemical properties gradually change from solid state to molecular elocali with decreasing particle size. The reasons for this elocali can be elocalize as two basic phenomena:

- Increase in surface-to-volume ratio
- Size quantization effect

Increase in Surface-to-volume Ratio

Owing to their small dimensions, the surface-to-volume ratio increases and number of surface atoms may be higher than those located in the crystalline lattice core. When no other molecules are adsorbed onto the nanocrystallites, the surface atoms are highly unsaturated and their electronic contribution to the elocali of the particles is totally different from that of the inner atoms. These effects may be even more marked when the surface atoms are ligated. This leads to different electronic transport properties, which account for the catalytic properties of the nanocrystalline particles.

Size Quantization Effect

Completely, an electronic effect that occurs in bulk metal and semiconductor to nanoparticles is described as the band structure gradually evolves with increasing particle size, *i. e.*, molecular orbital convert into delocalized band states.

The quasi-continuous density of states in the valence and the conduction bands splits into discrete electronic levels, the spacing between these levels and the band gap increasing with decreasing particle size **(Fig. 10)**.

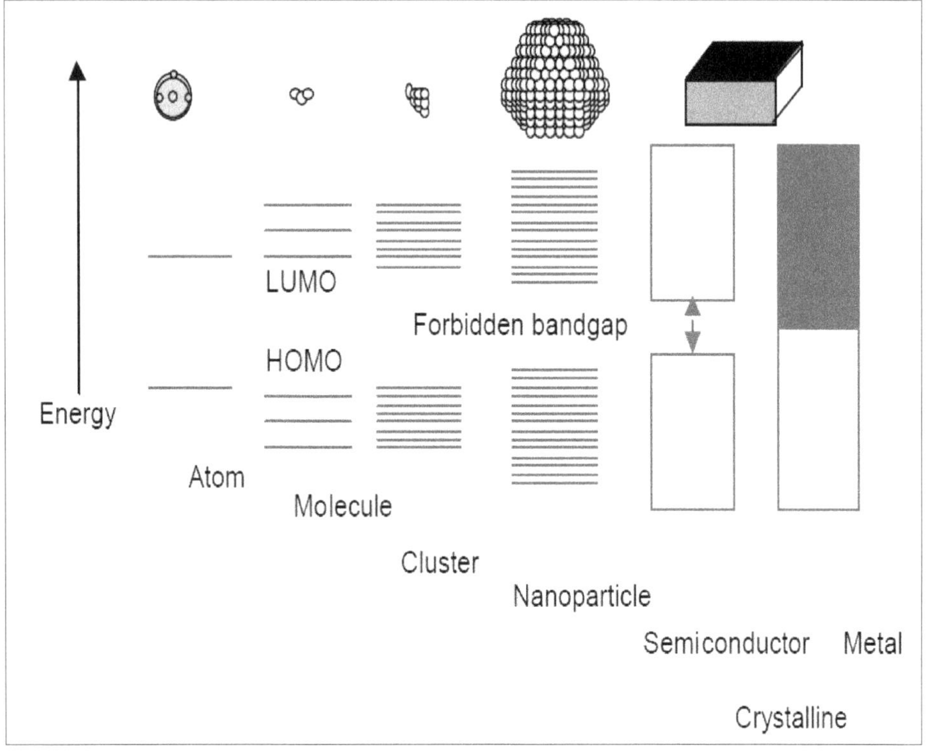

Fig. 10

The band gap increases when the particle size is decreased and the energy bands gradually convert into discrete molecular electronic levels. If the particle size is less than the De Broglie wavelength ($\lambda = h/p$ or h/mv) of the electrons, the charge carriers may be treated quantum mechanically as "particles in a box", where the size of the box is given by the dimensions of the crystallites. In semiconductors, the quantization effect is observed for clusters ranging from 1 nm to almost 10 nm. Metal particles consisting of 50 to 100 atoms with a diameter between 1 and 2 nm start to loose their metallic behavior and tend to become semiconductors. Particles that shows *size quantization effect* are called *Q-particles* or *quantum dots*.

Magic numbers: In semiconductor nanoparticles such as CdS, the growth of the initially formed smallest particles with an agglomeration number k occurs by combination of the particles. Thus, particles so formed would have the agglomeration number of 2*k*, 3*k* and so on. Metals have a cubic or hexagonal close-packed structure consisting of one central atom, which is surrounded in the first shell by 12 atoms, in the second shell by 42 atoms, or in principle by $10n^2+2$ atoms in the *n*th shell. *e.g.*: Most famous ligand stabilized metal clusters is a gold particle with 55 atoms (Au55) first reported by G. Schmid in 1981.

Quantum Confinement and Conductance

The conductance **G = I /V**, is the ratio of the total current **I** to the voltage drop **V** across the sample of length **l** in the direction of current flow. The quantum confinement of a carrier in a strip of width **w** leads to the discretization of energy levels given by

$$\epsilon_n = n^2h^2/(8m^*w^2).$$

Where ϵ_n is the energy of discrete energy levels; n is the principle quantum numer; h is the Plancks constant, m^* is the mass of electron and w is the nanostrip dimension.

Carbon Nanotube Bio-electronics Applications

Carbon nanotubes (CNTs) are allotropes of carbon. These cylindrical carbon molecules have interesting properties that make them potentially useful in many applications in nanotechnology, electronics, optics, biosensors and other fields of materials science, as well as potential uses in architectural fields (Fig 11 a & b). They exhibit extraordinary strength and unique electrical properties, and are efficient conductors of heat. Their final usage, however, may be limited by their potential toxicity.

Types: Single Wall CNT (SWCNT) & Multiple Wall CNT (MWCNT).

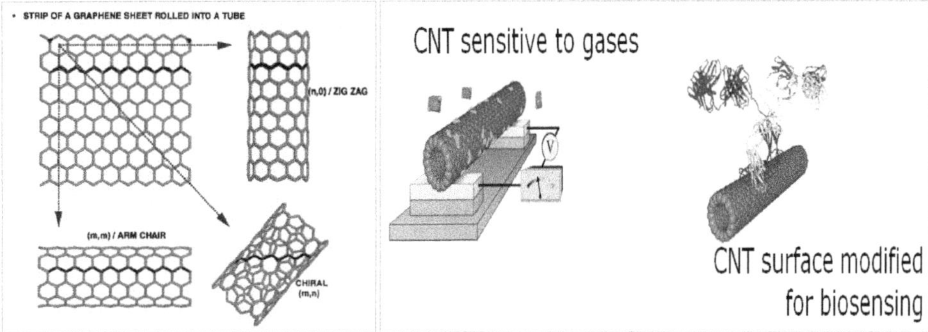

Fig 11 a & b

If the nanotube structure is armchair then the electrical properties are metallic. If the nanotube structure is chiral then the electrical properties can be either semiconducting with a very small band gap, otherwise the nanotube is a moderate semiconductor. In theory, metallic nanotubes can carry an electrical current density of 4×10^9 Amp/cm^2 which is more than 1,000 times greater than metals such as copper. Carbon nanotubes have potential applications for biosensors, sensing dangerous gases, studying proteins, *etc.*

Carbon Nanotube Devices

The carbon nanotubes are grown on silicon wafers by chemical vapor deposition (CVD). Lithographically-deposited electrodes allow us to fabricate nanotube wires **(Fig. 12)** and transistors.

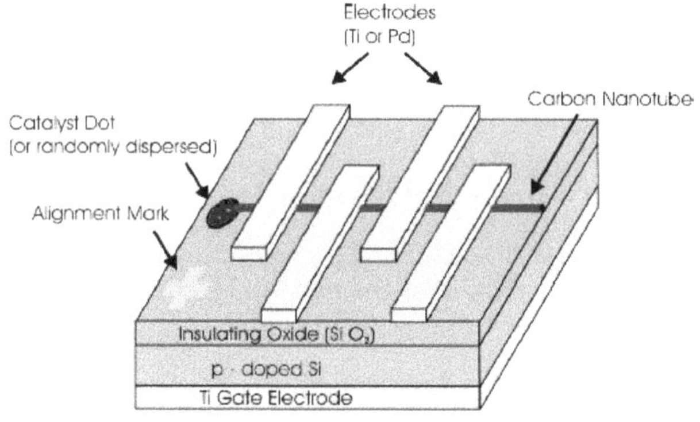

Fig. 12

Optical Properties of Nanomaterials

Nanoparticles are different from bulk materials and isolated molecules because of their unique optical, electronic and chemical properties. As the dimensions of the material is reduced, the electronic properties change drastically as the density of states and the spatial length scale of the electronic motion are reduced with decreasing size. Gold nanoparticles were used as a pigment of ruby-colored stained glass dating back to the 17th century. The bright red and purple colors are due to gold nanoparticles used in the Rose Window of the Cathedral of Notre Dame **(Fig. 13 a).** Lycurgus cup appears green in reflected light, but appears red when light is shone from inside, and is transmitted through the glass **(Fig. 13 b).**

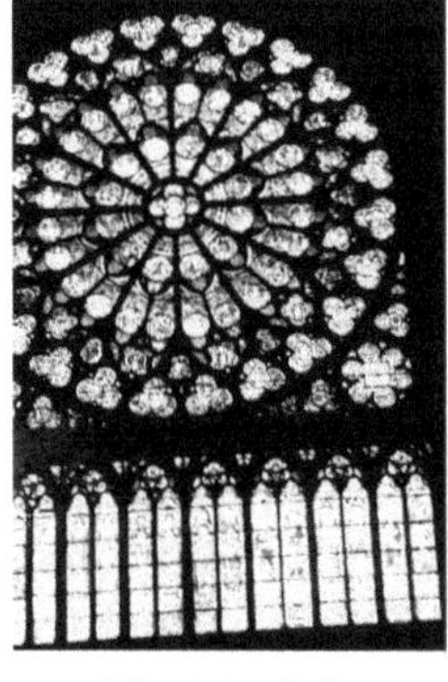

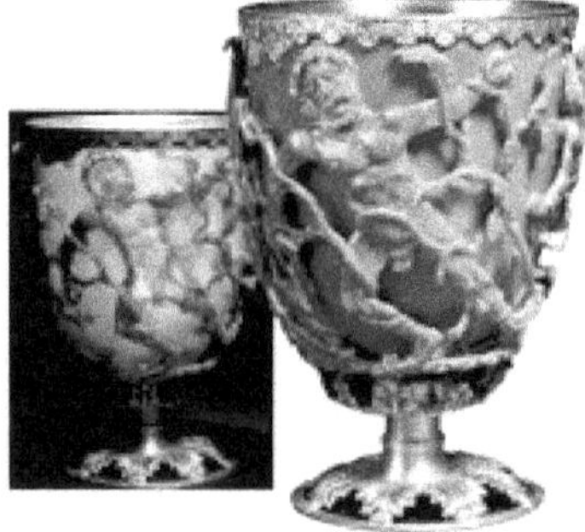

Surface Plasmons in gold nanoparticles

Fig. 13 a & b

A Surface Plasmon (SP) is a natural oscillation of the electron gas inside a gold nanosphere. SP frequency depends on the dielectric function of the gold, and the shape of the nanoparticle.

Surface Plasmon Resonance (SPR)

When a nanoparticle is much smaller than the wave length of light, coherent oscillation of the conduction band electrons induced by interaction with an electromagnetic field. This resonance is called Surface Plasmon Resonance (SPR) **(Fig.3.14).**

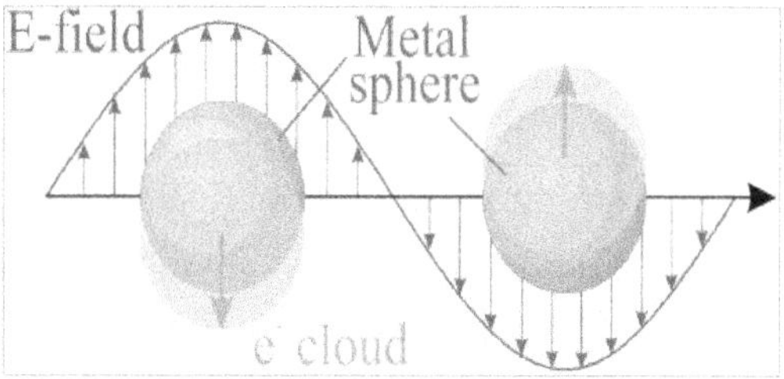

Fig. 14

Plasmon oscillation for a sphere, showing the displacement of the conduction electron charge cloud relativeto the nuclei.

The changes gold–blue–purple–red are largely geometric ones that can be explained with Mie theory, which describes light-scattering by a sphere. When the metal nanoparticle is larger than the ~30 nm, the electrons oscillating with the light is not perfectly in phase. Some electrons get behind; this phenomenon is called retardation effect or phase retardation. The subsequent changes, reddish – brown to orange to colorless, are due to quantum size effects. Each of the different sized arrangement of gold atoms absorbs and reflects light differently based on its energy levels, which are determined by size and bonding arrangement (Fig. 3.15). This is true for many materials when the particles have a size that is less than 100 nanometers in at least one dimension.

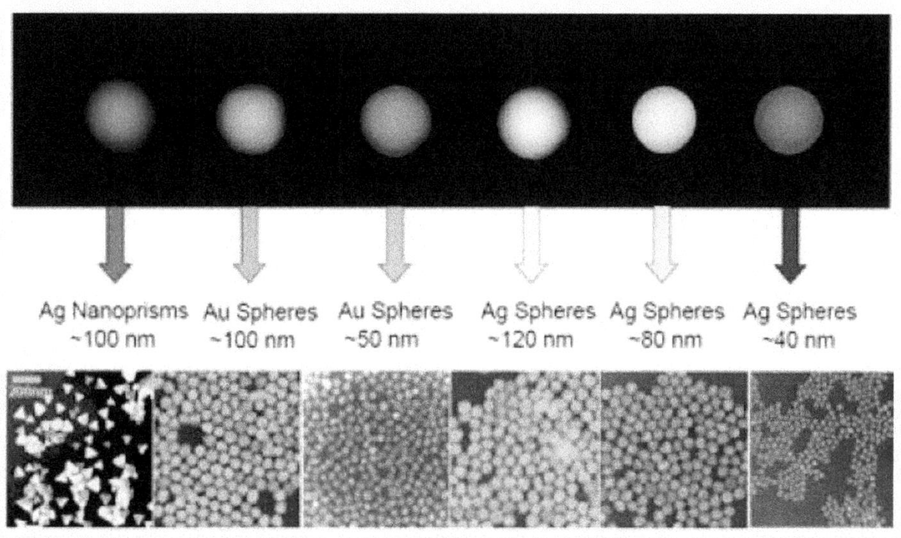

Fig. 15 **[www.ttu.ee]**

Self-assessment Questions

1. The CNTs are grown on __________ wafers by chemical vapor deposition. (Silicon)
2. __________is the characteristic of material remain deformed after the force is removed. (Plasticity)
3. Strain is a measure of amount of ___________ (deformation).
4. ____________model states that the smaller the grain size results in stronger the material (Hall Petch).
5. Energy required to create the unit area of new surface is ___________ (Surface energy)
6. Giant magnetoresistance is the application of _________ nanoparticles (super-paramagnetic)
7. SPR occurs when the size of metal particle is smaller than _______of light (wave length).

4

Physical Synthesis of Nanomaterials

Dr S Marimuthu

Nanotechnology is the study of engineering of materials with novel properties through controlled manipulation, synthesis and assembly of the material at the nanoscale level. Nanotechnology aims primarily on the synthesis of nanomaterials with desired stability. There are two main approaches to synthesize nanomaterial or nanoparticle. One is top-down approach and another one is the bottom-up approach. A top down approach where nanoparticles are synthesized by etching out crystals planes from bulk materials. Breaking down of the bulk material into nano sized structures or particles are top down approach (Etching and Ball milling) which are then subsequently assembled into nanomaterials. Bottom up approach involves self-assembly and coalescence of atoms, which gives rise to crystal planes, resulting in the formation of nanoparticles. The physical forces, which operates at nanoscale, combine atoms into larger stable structures (Fig 1). Chemical and biological synthesis of nanomaterials follow the bottom up approach.

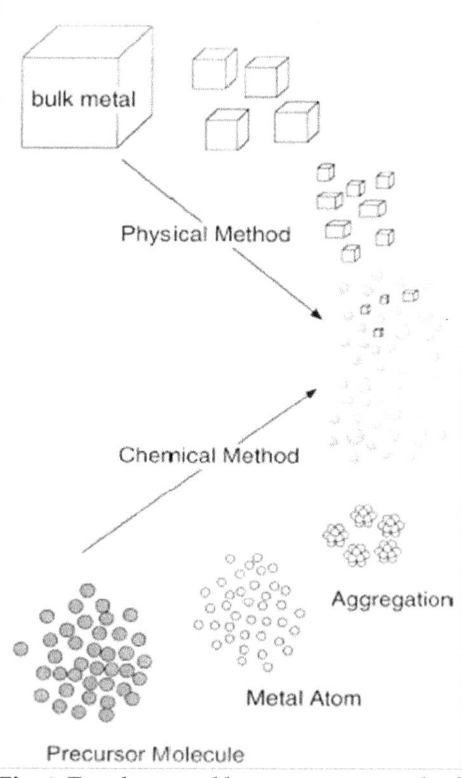

Fig. 1: Top down and bottom up approach of synthesizing nanomaterials

The bottom-up approach is more advantageous for producing nanoparticles with fewer defects and is more homogenous in nature whereas the imperfection of surface structure and significant crystallographic damage to the processed nanoparticles are common in top down approach. The bulk production of nanomaterials are possible in top down approach, but it involves higher machine costs and cross contamination while synthesis is possible. Production rates of nano particles through bottom up approach is very less, however, the processing time is to long. Synthesis of nanomaterials are classified into physical, chemical and biological methods based on the source of energy used during the synthesis, nature of chemical reaction and source of raw materials. Thid chapter discusses about the physical methods of synthesizing nanomaterials.

Physical Methods

Physical methods involves the use of mechanical energy, high energy radiations, thermal energy or electrical energy to effect material abrasion, melting, evaporation or condensation there by resulting in the synthesis of nanoparticles. The physical methods admire top-down strategy and are advantageous as the methods are free of solvent contamination. This method is simple to produce uniform monodispersed nanoparticles. The cross contamination and production of abundant waste materials are limitations of physical synthesis of nano particles. Laser ablation, electro spraying, inert gas condensation, physical vapour deposition, laser pyrolysis, flash spray pyrolysis, molecular beam epitaxy, high energy ball milling, melt mixing are some of the commonly used physical methods for synthesizing nano particles.

Physical Vapor Deposition

In general, deposition of gaseous materials over a substrate is referred as Vapor Deposition, which is further classified into physical and chemical vapor deposition. Physical Vapor Deposition is a coating process, involving the conversion of solid material into a gaseous phase by physical processes, which is then deposited on a substrate with some modification. The deposition of material over a wafer (substrate) is typically in the range of few nanometers to several micrometers. Physical vapor deposition involves physical removal of molecules or atoms from a source by evaporation or sputtering, which are transported through a vacuum or partial vacuum by the energy of the vapor particles, and condensed as a thin film on the surfaces of substrates.

The basic steps involved in physical vapor deposition are converting metal from solid to vapor phase (by either melting and evaporation or direct sublimation); transporting vapor phase material to the substrate and condensing gaseous material on substrate through nucleation and growth. Physical vapor deposition methods transfer kinetic energy to atoms in a solid or liquid, which is sufficient to overcome their binding energy causing removal of atoms. Evaporation is also used to heat the source material directly (resistive) or indirectly (electron beam and laser) until atoms to vaporize from the target materials. Sputtering is a process of physical impacts transferring kinetic energy to atoms in a target to liberate from source materials. Most commonly used techniques in physical vapor deposition are Sputtering, Electron beam evaporation, Pulsed Laser Deposition,

Molecular Beam Epitaxy and Inert Gas Condensation. Physical vapor deposition techniques are carried out in a vacuum system to avoid uncontrolled oxidation of source materials (target material that is to be evaporated) and final product of deposition as well as that of components of the synthesis system. Atoms in the vapor phase from the source material do not collide with each other under vacuum prior to arrival at substrate for deposition, since mean free path of the particles increases in vacuum system. The transport of atoms or molecules from the source to the growth substrate is straightforward along the line of sight under vacuum conditions, and therefore the conformal coverage and a uniform film over a large area is possible.

Electron Beam Evaporation

Electron beam evaporation is a vacuum-based physical vapor deposition technique. Electron beam is used to evaporate the atoms from the source materials. Electron beam evaporation is a process of evaporating source material, which is to be deposited on the wafer (substrate) by using beam of electrons to evaporate the target materials. The electrons are created from cathode materials through a heating process.

The Electron beam evaporation consists of ingot, which is the source to be deposited, filament (source of electrons), magnet (to bend an electron beam and direct towards source) and wafer over which target material is deposited as thin film (Fig 2). The ingot is positioned at a positive potential ensuring that there is no chemical interactions between the filament and the ingot material, where the filament is kept out of sight. A magnetic field is used to bend and direct the electron beam from its source to the ingot location, where an additional electric field is used to steer the beam over the ingot surface allowing uniform heating. The chamber is maintained at vacuum @ 10^{-8} to 10^{-4}Torr, which is required for steering electrons properly over the source. The power requirement for this technique is high (D.C. power @ 10 to 30 kV).

The first stage of the technique is heating filament (mostly tungsten), which will produce a beam of electrons on excitation due to heating. This process is achieved through thermionic emission, which is a process of discharging of electrons from a heated material. The energy is applied to the filament, enough to overcome the attractive force that holds electrons together in the filament. Once the electrons are excited which move about randomly in the chamber

The second stage is heating ingots that are to be deposited, which is generally referred as an evaporant kept in water-cooled grate. The source of the heating is beam of electrons produced from filament. These electrons must have a specific path to achieve a direction so that to concentrate at a point over the ignots for effective heating. Excited electrons moverandomly in the high vacuum chambersbecause there is no force of attraction. Hence, pair of electro magnets are placed, to attract the electrons in desired direction and deflect the route of the beam of electrons towards the material to be evaporated. The material will be heated on exposure to the electron beam to reach the boiling point. Then the evaporant will be converted to vapor phase, which started moving towards the wafer, where it is condensed on the surface of the wafer (substrate).

To summarize electron beam evaporation technique, electron beam hits the target and heats the target material, which evaporates when temperature reaches above its boiling point. The evaporated material is then transported and condensed onto the substrate.

The advantage of the technique is high rate of film deposition with less surface damage from the impinging atom. The technique achieves high purity deposition (due to high vacuum) and avoids unintentional heating of wafer. Alloys are also evaporated by this technique from an alloyed evaporant to produce composite thin films of materials. The disadvantage of the technique is the production of X-rays during the electron beam evaporation.

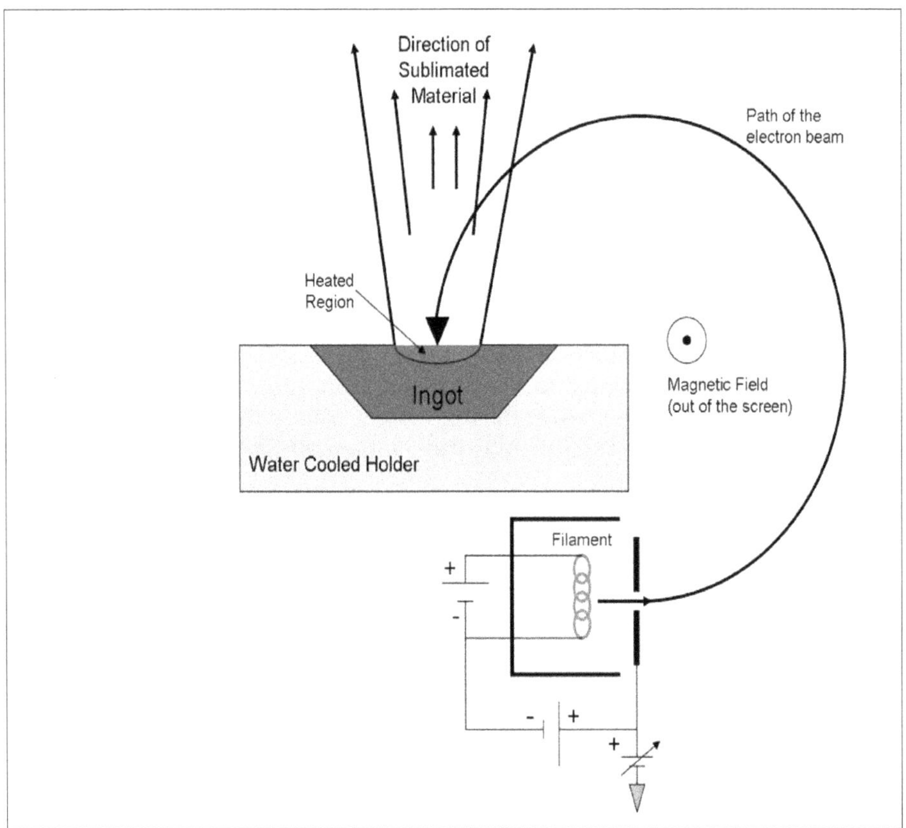

Fig. 2: Electron beam evaporation unit where ingot (evaporant) is positioned over hearth with water cooling mechanism and filament is used to generate electrons directed through magnetic field to the ingot location

Laser Ablation

Laser ablation method uses energy from high power laser beam to evaporate particles from a solid source. Laser is used either continuously or pulsed mode for evaporating materials. A pulsed laser beam of 30 ns pulses with energy in the range of 0.1-1 J and a frequency of 1-20 Hz is focused onto the target during the synthesis of nanomaterials. Generally pulsed laser is employed to remove the material from the target. The laser pulses hit the surfaces of target (evaporant) leading to melting, followed by evaporation and ionization of the material. The evaporated materials (plasma plume) deposited onto the suitably positioned substrate (Fig3). If the power density of a laser beam is greater than ablation threshold material (minimum energy density for removal of material), the materials will be evaporated. Usually shorter wavelength lasers including ArF (Argon fluoride), KrF (Krypton fluoride) excimer lasers, and Nd:YAG (Neodymium-doped Yttrium Aluminium Garnet) lasers are used for pulsed laser deposition. The focus of laser over material cause extremely high heating rate of the target surface (10^8 K/s) due to irradiation. Pulsed Laser Deposition is used for the preparation of variety of materials including polymers, oxides, metallic systems, fullerenes, carbides, nitrides, etc.

The laser energy is transferred to the charge carriers of free electrons in the case of metals while valance electrons in semiconductors which gets excited to the conduction band. After a short time of carrier thermallization, the carriers start transferring their energy to the lattice via electron-phonon coupling. The deformation or displacement of crystal lattices of atoms from the equilibrium position is described as phonons. When electrons interact with displacements is referred to as electron phonon coupling. The laser continues to pass the energy into the material even after finishing charge carries transferred energy to the lattice during electron phonon coupling. This process results in laser energy being dissipated as heat, where the laser beam incident over the material's surface, resulting in melting of the material. The melting of materials has caused area of pronounced heat effect and mechanical cracks, and other defects. The ablated materials form plasma plume reaching substrate for deposition. To summarize, pulsed laser deposition involves laser absorption on the target surface followed by ablation of the target material and creation of a plasma, sustainability of plasma, deposition of ablated materials along with plasma on the substrate and nucleation and growth of thin film over the substrate (wafer).

Pulsed laser deposition is a simple technique that requires the adjustment of laser power density and pulse repetition rate for the deposition. The process achieves multi-layered films of different materials by sequential ablation. The laser ablation technique produces film thickness of atomic monolayer over substrate. The most important feature of the technique is the retention of stoichiometry of the target in the deposited films.

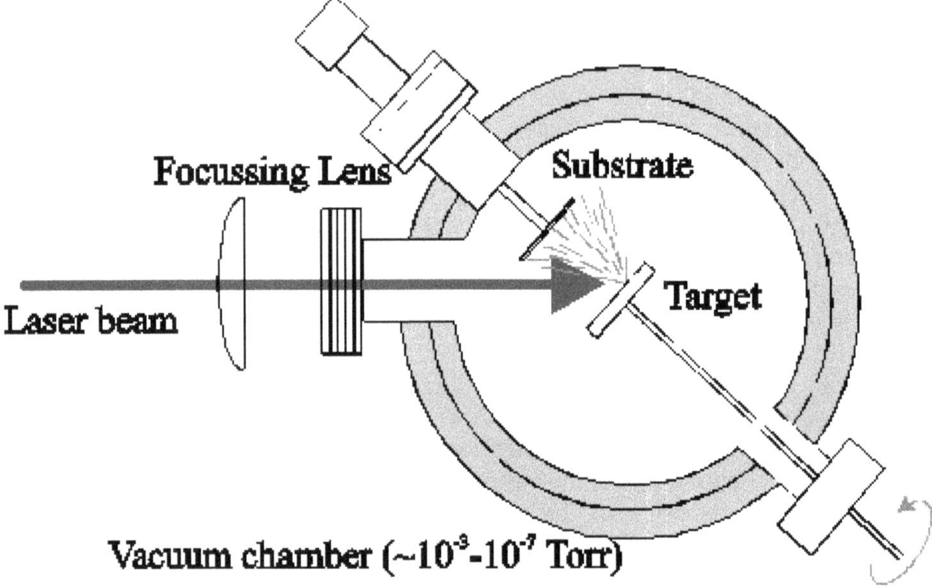

(Adopted from www1.phys.vt.edu accessed on 22nd September 2017)

Fig. 3: Pulsed laser ablation unit is carried out in vacuum chamber (10^{-3} to 10^{-2} torr) where laser is focused to target materials through focusing lenses.

Inert Gas Condensation

Inert gas evaporation–condensation technique synthesizes nanoparticles through the evaporation of a metallic source in an inert gas. This technique involves heating of target materials either through resistive heating or indirect heat (electrons and laser) until evaporation, an inert gas or reactive gas for collisions with material vapors, a cold finger on which clusters or nanoparticles are condensed, a scraper to scrape the nanoparticles and piston-anvil for compacting nanoparticles (Fig 4). The Insert gas condensation technique is the only technique which produces nanoparticles as end product.

Initially, the chamber is evacuated to a pressure of about 2×10^{-6} Torr by operating an oil diffusion pump. Metals or metal oxides are evaporated or sublimated by placing in boat of refractory metals like tungsten (W), tantalum (Ta) and Molybdenum (Mo). The temperature is set at a predetermined value for initial evaporation of materials. After evacuation, an inert gas (Helium, Xenon, or Argon) is back filled into the chamber at a low pressure, usually 0.5– 4.0 Torr, and the boar is heated rapidly (at constant temperature and inert gas pressure). On evaporation of source materials, the particles of small size (<5nm) are formed near the vicinity of source materials which in turn interact with other develops into bigger sized particles. The formed particles are removed from the source by forcing the inert gas. The rate of evaporation and gas pressure in the chamber determine the particle size and distribution. The evaporated cluster of particles colloid with inerts gas molecules forming bigger sized molecules over gas molecules and condensed over cold finger. On reaching the cold finger, inert gas molecules escape and reach gaseous phase of the chamber. If reactive gases like oxygen, hydrogen and ammonia are used instead of inert gases in the chamber, it will result in oxide, hydride and nitride particles. Clusters of nanoparticles are condensed on the cold finger (water or liquid nitrogen cooled) are scraped off inside the vacuum system, which fall through a funnel in the collection chamber where piston anvil mechanism helps to pelletize the collected particles.

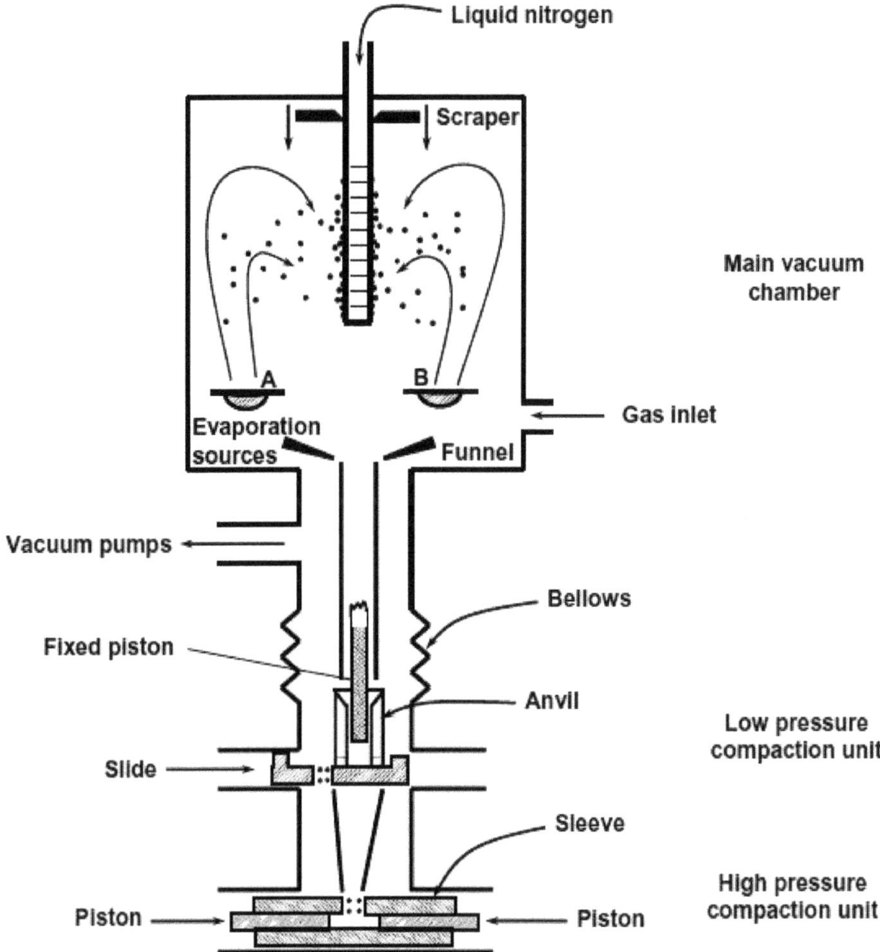

Fig. 4: Inert Gas Evaporation and Condensation unit for the synthesis of nanoparticles.

A wide range of nanoparticles including metals, alloys, intermetallic compounds, ceramics, semiconductors, and composites are synthesized through inert gas condensation technique, which is flexible technique for controlling the size and size distribution of the clusters/nanoparticles. The inert gas condensation produces nanoparticles with clean surfaces free from contamination. The possibilities for reacting, mixing, and coating various types, sizes, and morphologies source materials helps to synthesize new versatile materials. The technique is a continuous process, where scraping and compaction are carried out under ultra high vacuum conditions, and hence highest purity is maintained. The inert gas condensation technique allows *in-situ* diagnostics in the system Agglomeration is a problem in the inert gas condensation technique which is also costly process because it requires ultra high vacuum throughout the synthesis. Ensuring repeatability of parameters for the synthesis of nanoparticles and scaling up the process are difficult in the technique.

Sputtering

Sputtering is a thin film deposition technique, especially for retaining the composition of the original target material in the thin film (stoichiometric thin films). Sputtering is a process whereby particles are ejected from a solid target material due to bombardment of the target by energetic particles. The process is carried out by bombarding the surface of the target with gaseous ions under high voltage acceleration. In sputter deposition, usually Ar^+ ions are incident on a target at a high energy. The ionized inert gas molecules on interaction with target material may become neutral at the surface but due to their energy, incident ions may get implanted, get bounced back, create collision cascades in target atoms thus sputtering out target atoms/molecules.

Sputtering is carried out using Direct Current (DC) sputtering, Radio Frequency (RF) sputtering or magnetron sputtering. The mechanism of sputtering is using discharge or plasma of inert gas atoms or reactive gases to remove atoms or molecules physically from the target materials through the momentum transfer from ions into the target materials. The sputtering is carried out in a high vacuum or ultra high vacuum system equipped with electrodes of which one of them is sputter target and the other is a substrate, gas introduction (Fig 5).

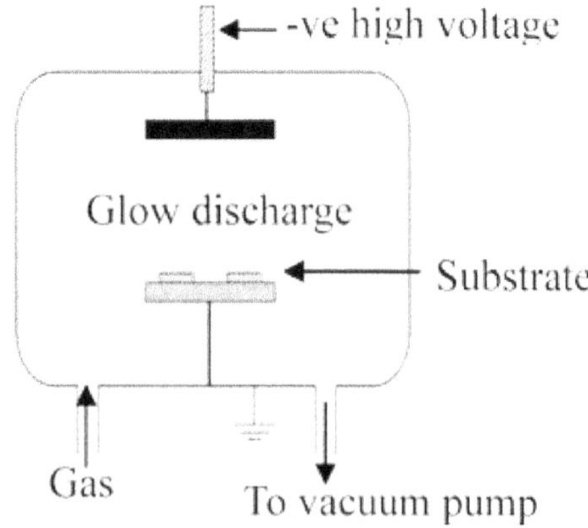

Fig. 5: DC sputtering for thin film deposition

Direct Current Sputtering

Direct sputtering, in which sputter target is held at high negative terminal while substrate is maintained at positive potential and grounded. The required base pressure is <10 P in the chamber where argon gas is introduced. A visible glow is observed when electrodes are biased, is called plasma (a mixture of electrons, ions, neutral atoms and photons released in various collisions). When sufficiently large number of ions is generated, this will be used to sputter off the target.

Sputtering is effective in producing non-porous compact films and multilayer films for mirrors or magnetic films for spintronics applications. Virtually any materials can be deposited by sputtering, since the coating material is passed into the vapor phase mechanically rather than through chemical or thermal process. Argon is usually used as a sputtering gas.

High Energy Ball Milling

The reduction of particle size by high energy ball milling is termed as mechanical milling which is a top down approach. John Benjamin developed mechanical milling in 1970, who used the technique to synthesize oxide dispersion strengthened (ODS) Nickel based alloys to withstand high temperature and pressure. High energy ball milling is one of the simplest ways of making nanoparticles of metals and alloys in the form of powder. The objective of milling is to reduce the particle size and blending of particles in new phases. The ball milling uses balls to impact upon the powder where balls fall freely and impact the powder.

Nanomaterials formed through a mechanical device, are referred as a mill, where the energy is imparted to a course-grained material to effect a reduction in particle size. The process of mechanical attrition of bulk materials through mechanical devices is called milling. Coarse-grained materials (usually metals but also ceramics and polymers) in the form of powders, are crushed mechanically in rotating drums by hard steel or tungsten carbide balls, under controlled atmospheric condition Mechanical deformation under shear conditions and high strain rates leads to the formation of nanostructures, where in energy is being continuously pumped into crystalline structures to create lattice defects.

The mechanism in mechanical milling is the ball-powder-ball collision, where powder particles are trapped between the colliding balls during milling and undergo de-formation and/or fracture processes which define the ultimate structure of the powder. The series of steps during high energy ball milling are powder mixture placed in the ball mill is subjected to high-energy collision from the balls (milling media) and high energy milling causes the structural disintegration of coarse-grained structure due to plastic deformation. High energy milling consists of repeated deformation (welding, fracturing and re-welding) of powder particles under a protective atmosphere. High energy milling induces structural changes and chemical reactions at room temperature due to mechanical energy rather than thermal energy.

The first stage of ball milling starts with compaction followed by the rearrangement and restacking of particles, producing some fine and irregularly shaped particles. The second stage of compaction involves elastic and plastic deformation of particles. The third stage involves particle fracture, and resulting in deformation and/or fragmentation of the particles.

The processes that define the milling are flattening of the elemental grains by plastic deformation followed by welding of elemental grains. Then formation of equilibrium size grains with parallel lamellae as a result of competition between welding and fracture processes occur followed by randomization of lamellae orientation as a result of repeated fracture and welding. Further refinement into grain microstructure takes place during the final stage of milling.

There are many types of mills such as planetary, vibratory, rod, tumbler mills etc. Two types of ball mill, the attritor and the horizontal ball mill are commonly used for the preparation of large quantities of material. The attritor consists of a stationary vertical cylindrical chamber, where the powder to be milled is placed along with the grinding medium (typically hardened steel balls). The powder and balls are agitated by rotating impellers. The attritors produce moderate quantities of material in moderate milling times. The horizontal ball mill, consists of a large (typically 1 m diameter) chamber that is rotated on a horizontal axis at a frequency slightly less than the critical frequency at which the balls are pinned to the inner wall of the chamber. The horizontal ball mill produce large quantities but the milling times are quite long.

The planetary ball mill and the vibratory ball mill are used extensively for ball milling in the research environment. The planetary ball mill utilizes two (or more) small counter-rotating vials located near the perimeter of a turntable. The planetary ball mill owes its name to the planet-like movement of vials. The vials are arranged on a rotating support disk, and a special drive mechanism causes them to rotate around their own axes (rotary motion around the mill axis and a planetary motion around the vial axis). The centrifugal force produced by the vials rotating around their own axes and the rotating support disk both act on the vial contents, consisting of material to be ground and the grinding balls. The vials and the supporting disk rotate in opposite directions, the centrifugal forces alternately act in like and opposite directions. This causes the grinding balls to run down to the inside of the vial causings the friction effect and followed by grinding of materials (Fig 6)', The vibratory ball mill where the vibrations are experienced in all three directions for milling. The most commonly used vibratory ball mill is the SPEX Model 8000.

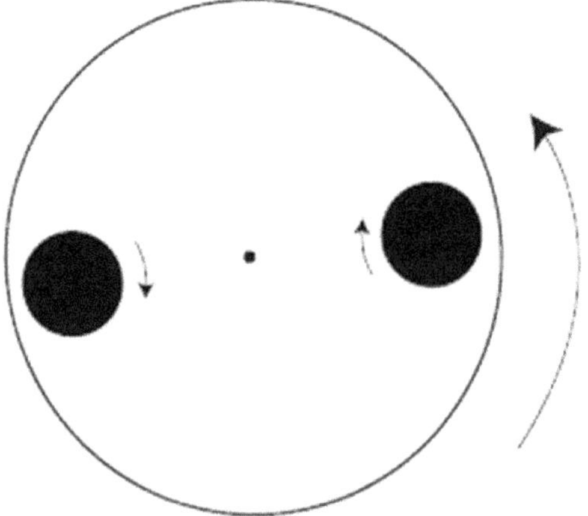

Fig. 6: Illustration on the illustration of planetary ball mill

The high specific gravity and larger balls give better milling because of high impact forces on the powders. However, the balls should be denser than the material to be milled. The highest collision energies are obtained if balls of different diameters are used for milling. The use of same sized milling balls produce tracks and consequently, the balls roll along a well-defined trajectory instead of hitting the end surfaces randomly. The ball to powder ratio (BPR) or charge ratio ranges from values as low as 1:1 to as high as 220:1 and usually it is 10:1 for planetary mills. The filling in the container is about 50 per cent of the volume of the chamber. The milling atmosphere contaminates the powder and hence milling is carried out in argon, or helium charged milling chambers. Contamination is avoided by milling the powders with a milling media made up of the same material as that of the powders being milled.

When mixture of powders (of different metals or alloys/compounds) are milled together, during which material transfer is involved to obtain a homogeneous alloy is mechanical alloying. Mechanical Milling refers to grinding of uniform composition powders, such as pure metals, intermetallics, or pre-alloyed powders, where material transfer is not required for homogenization. Mechanical milling requires half the time required for mechanic alloying to achieve the same effect.

Self-assessment Questions

Fill in the blank

1. ____________________ invented mechanical milling
2. ____________________ gas commonly used in the sputtering deposition technique
3. ____________________ laser used for laser ablation technique
4. ____________________ are refractory metals used for making boats for keeping source
5. ____________________ mills used for making nanoparticles at larger scale.

Short answers

6. Define physical vapor deposition
7. Define sputtering
8. Illustrate on the electron beam evaporation for the synthesis of nanomaterials
9. Differentiate sputtering and thermal evaporation
10. Define mechanical milling
11. Describe mechanism involved in size of reduction of bulk materials during milling.
12. Differentiate mechanical alloying and mechanical mixing.
13. Describe mechanism involved in the synthesis of nanoparticles during laser ablation.
14. Why vacuum is required in PVD technique during synthesis of nanoparticles?
15. Describe mechanism involved in Inert Gas Condensation with illustration.

5

Chemical Synthesis of Nanoparticles

Dr K. Raja and Dr K. Pandian

The particles in nanometer scale shows exciting optical and electronic characteristics when compared with respective bulk metals. Because of the inherent electronic properties of the metal and metal oxide nanoparticles these nanostructure materials are applied in various disciplines in recent days. Mostly these nanoparticles can be synthesized either top down or bottom up approaches. The conversion of bigger size particle or matter into tiny particles is called top down approach whereas smaller particles or atoms joined together forming particles in regular shape within nanometer scale dimension is called bottom up approach. The formation of nanoparticles by chemical reduction is an example for the later one and the reduction size with the help of mechanical crushing leads to the formation of fine nanoparticles is named as top down approach (Fig. 1). Mostly nanoparticles can be synthesized by chemical method because of easy to synthesis particles with uniform in size and high purity.

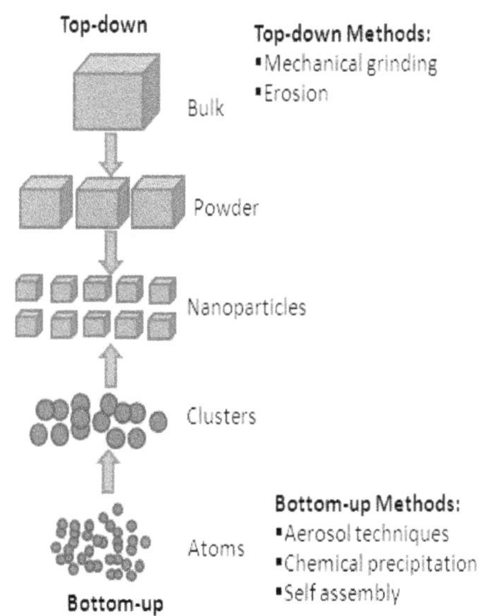

Fig. 1: Schematic diagram of top down and bottom up approaches

Chemical Methods

Chemical methods such as the reduction of transition metal salts are the most convenient ways to control the size of the particles. A key goal in the transition metal colloid area is the development of reproducible nano particles in opposition to traditional colloids. Generally nanoclusters should be or have at least (i) specific size (1-10 nm), (ii) well defined surface composition, (iii) reproducible synthesis and properties, and (iv) should be isolable and redispersible. Commonly, chemical synthesis is adopted for synthesizing nanoparticles as the method is easy where the size of the nanoparticles can be fine tuned by adjusting reaction environments such as altering the reducing agent concentration, reaction time, pH and temperature.

Principles: In most of the chemical synthesis process, the nanoparticles have been formed by the reduction and decomposition of precursors. There are two important processes are involved in the growth of nanocrystals from solution. First is the nucleation and second is the growth of the nanocrystals.

In a typical synthesis of nanocrystals, precipitation reaction is important to form the nanocrystals. The precipitation process involves nucleation step followed by crystal growth stages. Nucleation plays an important role in controlling the size and shape of the final product. Chemical colloidal nanocrystal synthesis involves the homogeneous nucleation occurs in the absence of a solid interface by combining solute molecules to produce nuclei.

The formation of nuclei can be described by LaMer diagram as shown in Figure 2. The process of nucleation and growth through the LaMer mechanism can be divided into three portions. (I) A rapid increase in the concentration of free monomers in solution, (II) the monomer undergoes "burst-nucleation" which significantly reduces the concentration of free monomers in solution. The rate of this nucleation is described as "effectively infinite" and after this point, there is almost no nucleation occurring due to the low concentration of monomers after this point; (III) following nucleation growth occurs under the control of the diffusion of the monomers through the solution.

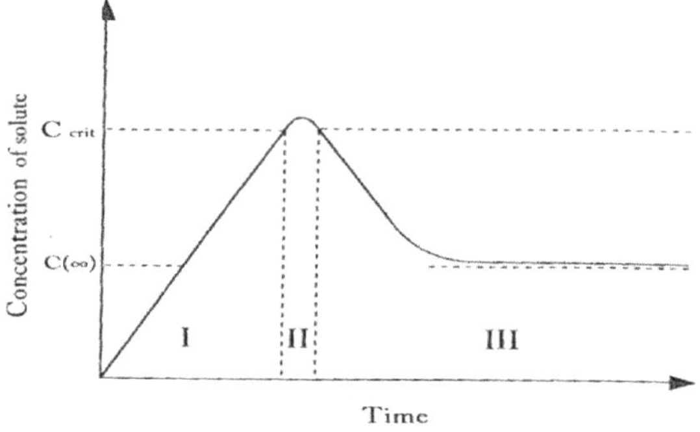

Fig. 2: Lamer's diagram (Lamer *et al.*, 1950)

Ostwald and Digestive Ripening: Ostwald ripening was first described in 1900. The mechanism of growth is caused by the change in solubility of NPs dependent on their size which is described by the Gibbs–Thomson relation. Due to the high solubility and the surface energy of smaller particles within solution, these redissolve and in turn allow the larger particles to grow even more. Digestive ripening is effectively the inverse of Ostwald ripening. Within this case, smaller particles grow at expense of the larger ones and have been described by Lee et al. where an applicable form of the Gibbs–Thomson equation, is derived. This process of formation is controlled once again by the surface energy of the particle within solution where the larger particle redissolves and in turn smaller particles grow.

The manipulation between thermodynamic and kinetic growth regimes is thus a critical factor in determining nanoparticle shape.The final nanoparticle morphology can be controlled by dictating the shape of nuclei and directing the growth of the nuclei or nanocrystals. Nuclei can take on a variety of shapes determined by the chemical potentials of the different crystallographic faces, which are in turn highly dependent on the reaction environment such as temperature and solute concentration. The nuclei shape can have a strong effect on the final nanocrystal shape, for example, through selected growth of high-energy crystal faces of the nuclei. In the presence of a surfactant in bulk solution, the products are capped by surfactant molecules, resulting in the restriction of the particle growth as well as the good dispersibility of the product in reaction solvent.

Two Step Mechanisms: The Finke-Watzky two step mechanism is a process of nucleation and growth where both steps happen simultaneously. The first is a slow continuous nucleation, and the second is the autocatalytic surface growth which is not diffusion controlled. This process was discovered through the reduction of transition metal salts by hydrogen which was studied by following the reduction of cyclohexene. Currently, this method is shown through the kinetic fitting of the cyclohexene reduction and has not been proven explicitly. Although, this method is different from classical nucleation, the nucleation step still follows a critical size described within a classical nucleation framework (Fig.4).

Methods of Chemical Synthesis

In chemical synthesis, there are different methods *viz.*, chemical vapour deposition, Co-precipitation, sol-gel, polyol, microemulsion, microwave assisted synthesis, photoreduction using gamma rays, ultrasonic waves, and liquid plasma, spray drying, spray pyrolysis, solvothermal synthesis, electrospinning and supercritical method are employed for synthesising nanoparticles/nanomaterials. In this chapter, sol–gel process, polyol, microwave assisted synthesis, electrospinning and microemulsion methods of NPs /nanoparticles are discussed.

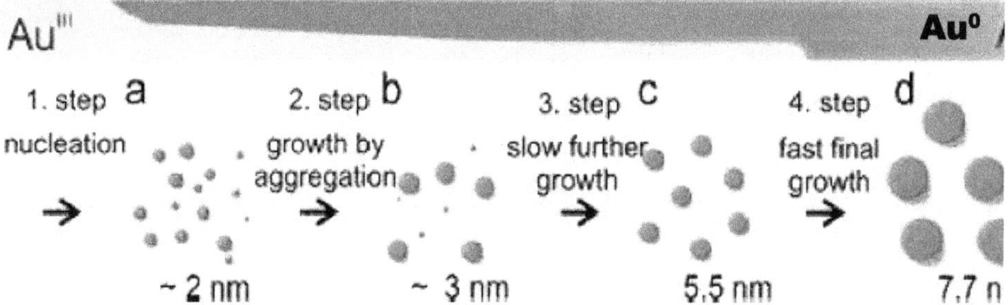

Fig. 3: Schematic diagram for the reduced process of gold nanoparticle formation reduction method (Nguen *et al.*, 1950)

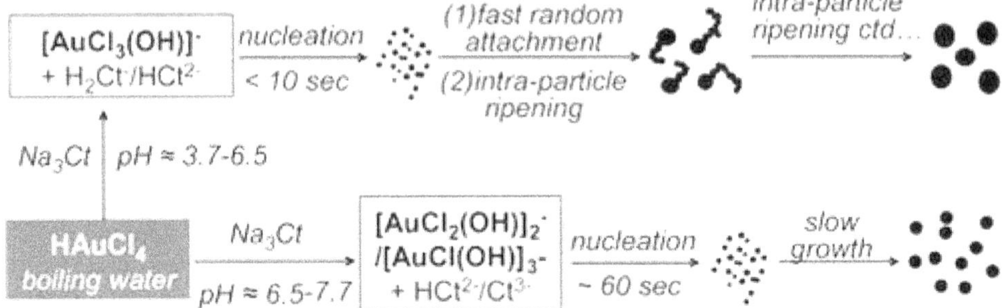

Fig. 4: Schematic diagram of two reaction pathways for the formation of gold nanoparticle by citrate reduction method (Nguen *et al.*, 1950)

Sol-gel Method

Sol–gel processing is a ***wet chemical*** and promising method for the preparation of nano dimensional materials. It is a very long known process since the late 1800s and the versatility of the technique has been rediscovered in the early 1970s when glasses were produced without high temperature melting process. Sol-gel is a chemical solution process used to make ceramic and glass materials in the form of thin films, fibers or powders. In this chemical procedure, the monomers are converted into colloidal solution (Sol) that gradually converted into a gel like diphasic system (integrated net work or gel), which contains both liquid phase and solid phase and the morphologies of these two phases range from discrete particles to continue polymer networks. Initially a significant amount of fluid may have to be removed from solution to recognize the gel like properties. Sol-gel method is a low temperature technique and moreover it is cheap. One of the advantages of this method is the ability to control the microstructure of final product by controlling chemical reaction parameters.

The precursor for synthesizing these colloids consists of ions of metal alkoxides and aloxysilanes. The most widely used are tetramethoxysilane (TMOS), and tetraethoxysilanes (TEOS) which form silica gels. Alkoxides are immiscible in water. They are organo metallic precursors for silica, aluminum, titanium, zirconium and many others. Mutual solvent alcohol is used. The sol gel process involves initially a homogeneous solution of one or more selected alkoxides. These are organic precursors for silica, alumina, titania, zirconia, among others. Sol-gel formation occurs in four stages.

Processes in Sol-gel process: There are three important steps namely hydrolysis, condensation, growth and agglomeration involved in Sol-gel process (Fig. 5).

Hydrolysis: The first step in a sol-gel reaction is the formation of an inorganic polymer by hydrolysis and condensation reactions, i.e., the transformation of the molecular precursor into a highly crosslinked solid. Hydrolysis leads to a sol, a dispersion of colloidal particles in a liquid. During hydrolysis, addition of water results in the replacement of (OR) group with (OH-) group. Hydrolysis can be accelerated by adding a catalyst such as HCl and NH_3. Hydrolysis continues until all alkoxy groups are replaced by hydroxyl groups

$$MOR + H_2O \rightarrow M\,OH + ROH$$

Condensation: Condensation results in a gel, an interconnected, rigid and porous inorganic network enclosing a continuous liquid phase. This transformation is called the sol-gel transition. Condensation reactions between two hydroxylated metal species. Aqueous Sol-Gel Chemistry leads to M-O-M bonds under release of water (oxolation), whereas the reaction between a hydroxide and an alkoxide leads to M-O-M bonds under release of an alcohol (alkoxolation).

$$MOH + ROM \rightarrow MOM + ROH$$

$$\text{or } MOH + HOM \rightarrow MOM + H_2O$$

Growth and Agglomeration

As the number of alkoxane bonds increase, the molecules aggregate in the solution, where they form a network, a gel is formed upon drying. The water and alcohol are driven off and the network shrinks. There are two possibilities to dry the gels. Upon removal of the pore liquid under hypercritical conditions, the network does not collapse and aerogels are produced. When the gel is dried under ambient conditions, shrinkage of the pores occurs, yielding a xerogel.

Advantages: One of the highly attractive features of the sol-gel process is the possibility to shape the material into any desired form such as monoliths, films, fibers, and monosized powders, and subsequently to convert it into a ceramic material by heat treatment.

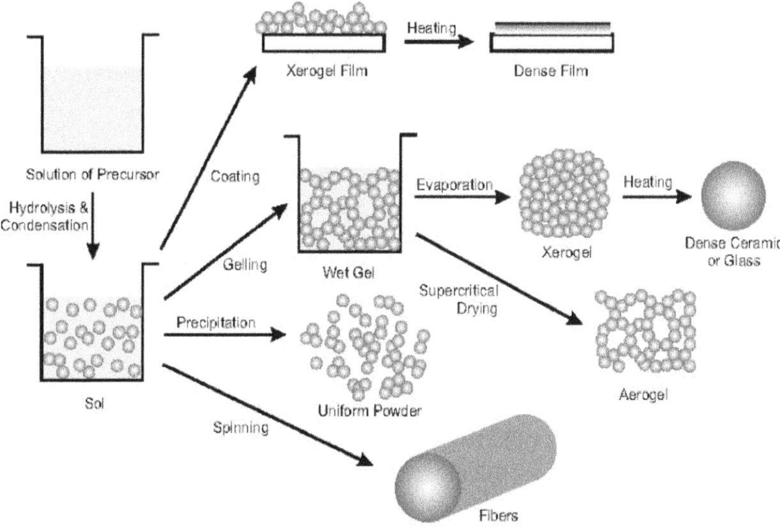

Fig. 5: Various steps in the sol-gel process to control the final morphology of product

Disadvantages: The aqueous chemistry of transition metal ions can be rather complicated because of the formation of a large number of oligomeric species, depending on the oxidation state and the pH or the concentration. The role of the counter anions, which are able to coordinate the metal ion giving raise to a new molecular precursor with different chemical reactivity towards hydrolysis and condensation, is almost impossible to predict. These ions can influence the morphology, the structure and even the chemical composition of the resulting solid phase. Also the removal of these anions from the final metal oxide product is often a problem.

Polyol Method of Nanoparticles Synthesis

The synthesis of metal-containing compounds in polyol (ethylene glycol) is defined as polyol synthesis of nanoparticles. In the polyol process, the polyol can be used as both the solvent and the reductant, therefore, in many cases; no additional reducing reagent is needed in the reaction system. In contrast, a reductant is usually necessary for the preparation of metal nanostructures in aqueous solution. When ethylene glycol is used as the solvent and reductant, metallic nanostructures (M) are produced by the following chemical reactions according to the reduction mechanism proposed by Fievet *et al.*(1987)

$$CH_2\,OH\text{-}\,CH_2\,OH \rightarrow CH_3\,CHO + H_2O$$

$$CH_3CHO + M^{n+} \rightarrow M\ CH\ COCOCH\ H\ O$$

Polyol method can be employed for the synthesis of relatively large Pt nanopowder (e.g. 5-13 nm) with high purity. The reduction is based on the decomposition of ethylene glycol and its conversion to diacetal. Alcohols such as methanol, ethanol or propanol work simultaneously as solvent and as reducing agents being oxidized to aldehydes or ketones.

$$\underset{OH}{CH_2}\!-\!\underset{OH}{CH_2} \xrightarrow{-H_2O} H_3C\!-\!CHO \xrightarrow{M(II)} H_3C\!-\!\underset{O}{\overset{\|}{C}}\!-\!\underset{O}{\overset{\|}{C}}\!-\!CH_3 + M_{(0)}$$

Refluxing metal salts or complexes such as H2PtC16, HAuC14, PdC12, RhC13 in an alcohol/water (1/1, v/v) mixture yields nanocrystalline metal powders in the absence of stabilizers. The homogeneous dispersion of colloidal nanoparticles can be obtained in the presence of protective polymers such as polyvinylpyrrolidone (PVP).

Microwave Assisted Synthesis of Nanoparticles

Microwaves are the electromagnetic waves with frequencies ranging from 0.3 to 300 GHz and with wavelengths of between 1 mm and 1 m, which are between infrared and radio frequency waves in the electromagnetic spectrum. The commonly used frequency in laboratories and homes for microwave heating is 2.45 GHz with a wavelength of about12.24 cm.

Microwave chemistry: Microwave chemistry is the science of applying microwave irradiation to chemical reactions. The basic principles of microwave chemistry have been focused mostly on the reaction engineering in the microwave field. The microwave heating involves two main mechanisms, **dipolar polarization and ionic conduction.** Microwaves generally heat any material containing mobile electric charges such as polar molecules or conducting ions in a solvent or in a solid. During the microwave heating, polar molecules such as water molecules try to orientate with the rapidly changing alternating electric field; thus heat is generated by the rotation, friction, and collision of molecules (dipolar polarization mechanism). In the case of ions, any ions present in solution will move through the solution based on the orientation of the electric field, and because this is in constant fluctuation, the ion is moving in constantly changing directions through the solution, causing a local temperature rise due to friction and collision. Semiconducting and conducting samples heat when ions or electrons within them form an electric current and energy is lost due to the electrical resistance of the material (ionic conduction mechanism) (Fig.6)

Microwave wave assisted methods have been employed for the convenient and reproducible synthesis of well-defined noble and transition core–shell metallic nanoparticles with tunable shell thicknesses. Micro wave heating provides superb value to the overall sustainable process development via process intensification including the flow systems. An example of NPs synthesis using microwaves is given below.

Microwave assisted ZnO NPs synthesis : In a typical synthesis process, a precursor salt of zinc nitrate (15mL of 1.6 mol L^{-1}) is diluted in deionized water (32mL) to obtain a Zn^{2+}solution. Afterwards, a base (4ml of 3.2 mol L^{-1}) Sodium hydroxide (NaOH) is added dropwise into the solution with magnetic stirring at room temperature to get a colloid system, which is maintained under stirring for 10min. Then, the reaction mixture is transferred into a vial and treated at selected

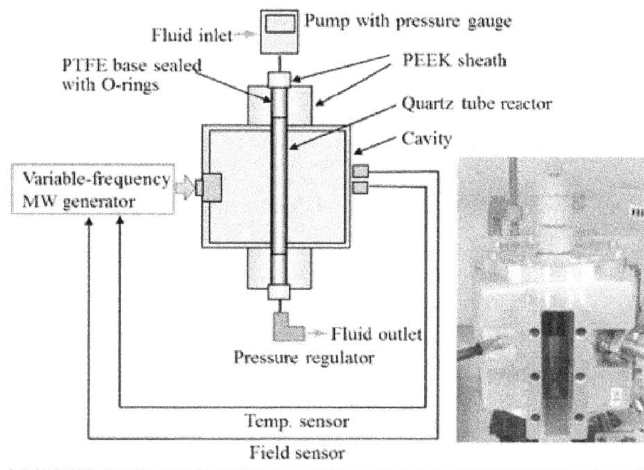

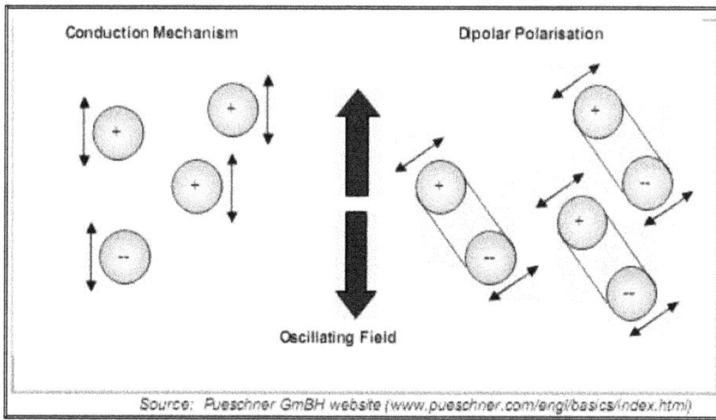

Fig. 6: Microwave apparatus set up and dipolar polarization and ionic conduction

temperature 140°Cfor specific time 20min. under temperature-controlled mode in a microwave accelerated reaction system. It must be mentioned that the system is programmed with a first temperature ramp where the target temperature is reached after 10min. When the reaction is finished, take the settled or precipitated particles and cool it at room temperature. The white precipitate is collected by filtration and washed with deionized water and ethyl alcohol for several times. Finally, the product is to be dried at 65°C in a vacuum oven for 3 h and characterize the particles with nanotechnology tools (Barreto *et al.*, 2013).

Electrospinning

Electrospinning, a broadly used technology for electrostatic fiber formation which utilizes electrical forces to produce polymer fibers with diameters ranging from 2nm to several micrometers using polymer solutions of both natural and synthetic polymers. Utility of this technique has been a tremendous increase in research and commercial attention over the past decade. This process offers unique capabilities for producing novel natural nanofibers and fabrics with controllable pore structure with smaller pores and higher surface area than regular fibers.

Electrospun fibers have been successfully applied in various fields, such as, nanocatalysis, tissue engineering scaffold, protective clothing, filtration, biomedical, pharmaceutical, optical electronics, healthcare, biotechnology, defense and security and environmental engineering. Overall, this is a relatively robust and simple technique to produce nanofibers from a wide variety of polymers.

Advantages

- High surface-to-volume ratio
- Tunable porosity
- Malleability to conform to a wide variety of sizes and shapes and the ability to control the nanofiber composition to achieve the desired results from its properties and functionality.

Electrospinning process : Electrospinning, a spinning technique, is a unique approach using *electrostatic forces* to produce fine fibers from polymer solutions or melts and the fibers thus produced have a thinner diameter (*from nanometer to micrometer*) and a larger surface area than those obtained from conventional spinning processes. Furthermore, a DC voltage in the range of several tens of kVs is necessary to generate the electrospinning. Various techniques such as electrostatic precipitators and pesticide sprayers work similarly to the electrospinning process and this process, mainly based on the principle that strong mutual electrical repulsive forces overcome weaker forces of surface tension in the charged polymer liquid (*Chew et al.*, 2006a). Currently, there are two standard electrospinning setups, vertical and horizontal. With the expansion of this technology, several research groups have developed more sophisticated systems that can fabricate more complex nanofibrous structures in a more controlled and efficient manner. Electrospinning is conducted at room temperature with atmosphere conditions. The typical set up of electrospinning apparatus is shown in Fig. 7 (a and b).

Components : Basically, the standard laboratory electrospinning system consists of three major components a spinneret (typically a hypodermic syringe needle) connected to a high-voltage (5 to 50 kV) direct current power supply, a syringe pump, and a grounded collector. A polymer solution, sol-gel, particulate suspension or melt is loaded into the syringe and this liquid is extruded from the needle tip at a constant rate by a syringe pump. Alternatively, the droplet at the tip of the spinneret can be replenished by feeding from a header tank providing a constant feed pressure. This constant pressure type feed works better for lower viscosity feed stocks.

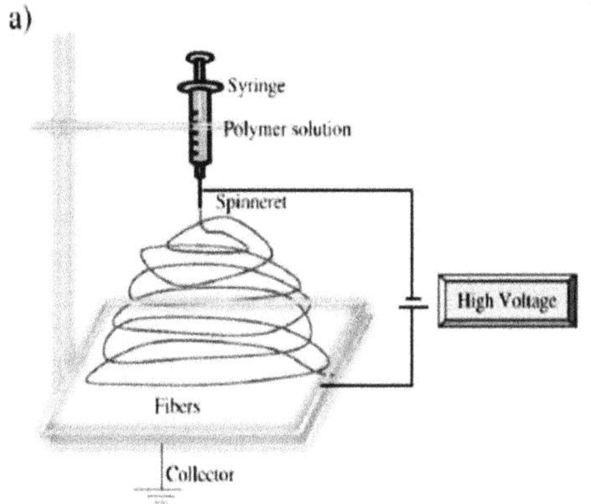

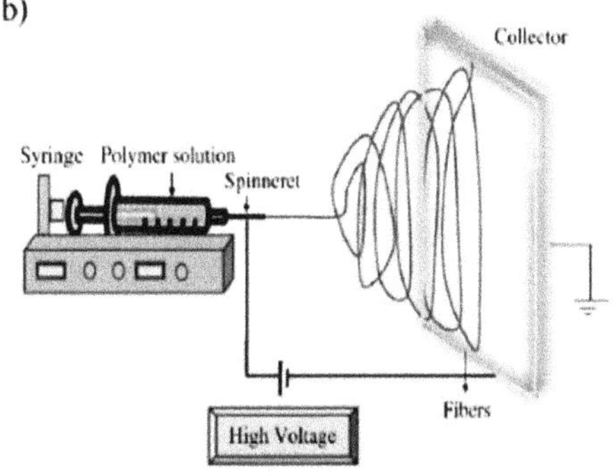

Fig. 7a &b. Electrospinning set up

In the electrospinning process, a polymer solution held by its surface tension at the end of a capillary tube is subjected to an electric field and an electric charge is induced on the liquid surface due to this electric field. When the electric field applied reaches a critical value, the repulsive electrical forces overcome the surface tension forces. Eventually, a charged jet of the solution is ejected from the tip of the Taylor cone and an unstable and a rapid whipping of the jet occurs in the space between the capillary tip and collector which leads to evaporation of the solvent, leaving a polymer behind. (Taylor, 1969; Yarin et al., 2001; Adomaviciute and Milasius, 2007). The jet is only stable at the tip of the spinneret and after that instability starts. Thus, the electrospinning process offers a simplified technique for fiber formation (Fig.8)

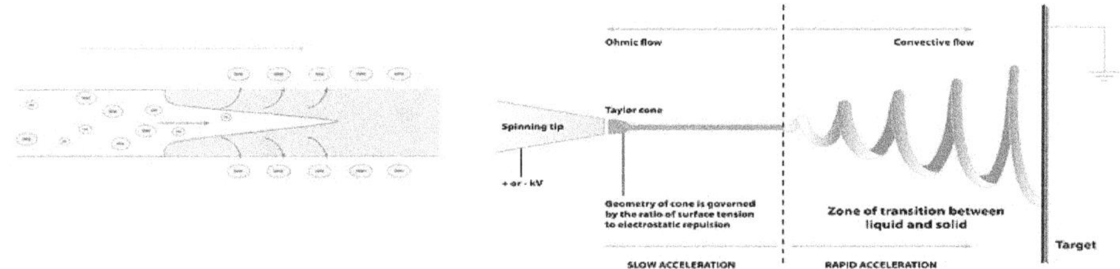

Fig. 8: Tayler cone and fibre formation by electrospinning

Polymers used in electrospinning : There are a wide range of polymers that used in electrospinning and are able to form fine nanofibers within the submicron range and used for varied applications. Electrospun nanofibers have been reported as being from various synthetic polymers, natural polymers or a blend of including proteins, nucleic acids and even polysaccharides.

Characterizations of electrospun nanofibers: Geometric properties of nanofibers include fiber diameter, diameter distribution, fiber orientation, and fiber morphology (e.g. cross-section shape and surface roughness) are characterized with SEM, field emission scanning electron microscopy (FESEM), transmission electron microscopy (TEM), atomic force microscopy (AFM) , XRD, FTIR and DSC

Applications: Recently, researchers have begun to look into various applications of electrospun fibers and mats as these provide several advantages such as high surface to volume ratio, very high porosity and enhanced physico-mechanical properties. Electrospun nanofibers are broadly applied in biomedical applications, as tissue engineering scaffolds, in wound healing, drug delivery, filtration, as affinity membrane, in immobilization of enzymes, small diameter vascular graft implants, healthcare, biotechnology, environmental engineering, defense and security, and energy storage and generation and in various researches that are ongoing.

Micro-emulsion Method

Micro-emulsions are complex liquids with potentials for current and future application prospects. They consist of oil, water, surfactant and co-surfactant that form a clear solution. The amphiphilic nature of a surfactant, such as cetyltrimethylammonium bromide (CTAB) as described later, makes them miscible with water and oil. Micro emulsions can be either 'water in oil' (w/o) or 'oil in water' (o/w) stabilized by surfactant molecules with morphologies similar to those of micelles and reverse micelles where the interfacial tension is extremely low

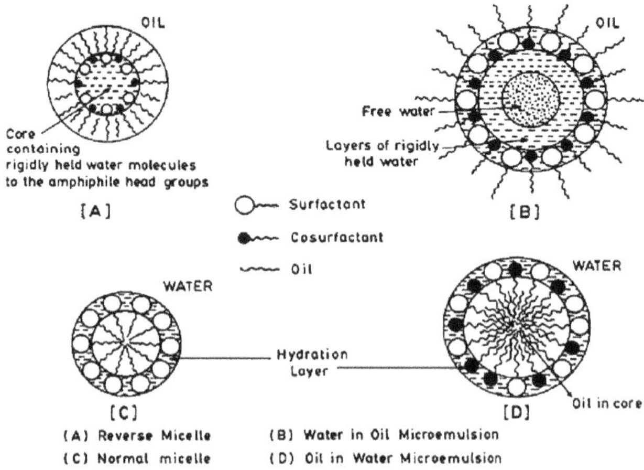

Fig. 9: Representations of reverse micelles and micro-emulsions

between the two phases. With these characteristics, micro-emulsions appear to be an ideal plat form to bring together the metal precursor (e.g. water-soluble) and the reactant (e.g.oil-soluble) to enable the reduction of the metal to occur. Generally, the size of micro emulsions is small and uniform. Hence, they can be regarded as a micro reactor for the synthesis of nanoparticles. As the water concentration alters, the system can change from a w/o to an o/w micro-emulsion, which is illustrated in. These systems offer a wide range of possibility and flexibility to carry out the synthesis (Fig. 9&10).

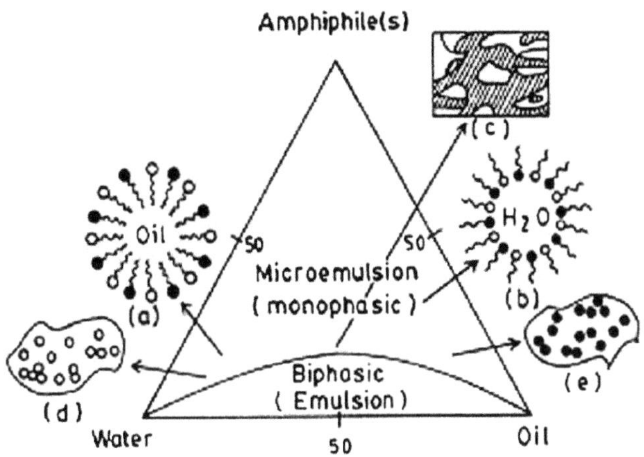

Fig. 10: A ternary phase diagram showing how various complexes depend on the different surfactants and intrinsic structures: (a) o/w micro-emulsion, (b) w/o micro-emulsion, (c) bicontinuous dispersion, (d) isolated and aggregated o/w dispersion, and (e) isolated and aggregated w/o dispersion

Influence of Reducing Agents in the Synthesis of Nanoparticles

The size and size distribution of metallic colloids vary significantly with the types of reduction reagents used in the synthesis. In general, a strong reduction reaction promotes a fast reaction rate and favours the formation of smaller nanoparticles. However, a slow reaction may result in either wider or narrower size distribution. If the slow reaction leads to continuous formation of new nuclei or secondary nuclei, a wide size distribution would be obtained. On the other hand, if no further nucleation or secondary nucleation occurs, a slow reduction reaction would lead to diffusion-limited growth of the nuclei would be controlled by the availability of the zero valent atoms. Metal nanoparticles have a tendency to agglomerate, and therefore, it is necessary to protect them using surfactants or polymers, such as cyclodextrin, PVP, PVA, citrate or quaternary ammonium salts

Using the same reduction reagent, nanoparticle size can be varied by changing the synthesis conditions. In addition, it was found that the reduction reagents have noticeable influences on the morphology of the gold colloidal particles. Gold particles with spherical shape were obtained using sodium citrate or hydrogen peroxide as reduction reagents, whereas faceted gold particles were formed within hydroxylamine hydrochloride and citric acid were used as reduction reagents. Furthermore, concentration of the reduction reagents and pH value of the reagents have noticeable influences on the morphology of the grown gold nanoparticles.

Advantages of Chemical Methods

- In chemical reduction method it is possible to fine tune the form (shape) and size of the nanoparticles by changing the reducing agent, the dispersing agent, the reaction time and the temperature.
- The chemical reduction method carries out chemical reduction of the metal ions to their 0 oxidation states (i.e., $M^{n+} \rightarrow M^{\circ}$); the process uses non-complicated equipment or instruments, and can yield large quantities of nanoparticles at a low cost in a short time.
- Stabilization of nanoparticles from agglomeration
- Extraction of nanoparticles from solvent
- Surface modification and application
- Processing control (Shape and size of the nanoparticles can be fine tuned by changing the reducing agent, the dispersing agent, the reaction time and the temperature) and
- Mass production.

Self-assessment Questions

1. What is bottom up approach of nanoparticles synthesis?
2. Substantiate why chemical synthesis is mostly used for nanomaterials fabrication.
3. Explain the significance of reducing agent in chemical synthesis of nanomaterials.
4. Describe the sol-gel and microwave synthesis of nanoparticles.
5. Explain the polyol method of NPs synthesis with example.
6. Elucidate the process in chemical reduction method of nanoparticle synthesis.
7. Write the principle of electrospinning.
8. What are the factors influencing the electrospinning of nanomaterial synthesis?
9. Describe the process of electrospinning of nanomaterial synthesis with illustration.
10. Explain the microemulsion technique of nanomaterials synthesis.
11. List the different chemical methods of nanomaterials synthesis.

Fill in the blanks

1. In chemical synthesis, NPs are synthesised by __________ and __________ process of precursors
2. __________ ripening explains the crystalline growth of NPs are synthesised in chemical method
3. ____________________ is used to protect the NPs from agglomeration
4. Wet chemical method of nanoparticles synthesis is ________________
5. Synthesis of metal-containing compounds in ethylene glycol is defined as____________________
6. The mechanisms of microwave heating are ________________ and ____________
7. Frequency of microwaves is ______________________________________
8. The voltage required to produce nanofibre in e-spin is ______________
9. Wave length of microwaves is ___________________________
10. In sol-gel method, the precursor for synthesizing NPs consists____________ and ____________ ions

6

Biological Synthesis of Nanoparticles Using Plants and Microorganisms

Dr Haripriya Shanmugam

Nanoparticles have been synthesized and used by humans for centuries. Currently, varieties of metal nanoparticles are utilized in nano-enabled devices, medical, food and agricultural products. As of date, biologically synthesized nanomaterials are predominantly metal nanoparticles. The journey of metal nanoparticles dates back to the famous Lycurgus cup to Michael faraday's gold colloids to current, cadmium sulfide quantum dots. It is well known that the optical, electronic, and catalytic properties of metal nanoparticles are greatly influenced by their size, shape, and crystal structure. Silver (Ag) and gold (Au) nanoparticles of different size and shapes possess unique optical scattering property. Thus, synthesis of metal nanoparticles with defined size and morphology gained much attention.

Conventionally, nanoparticles are synthesized through physical and chemical methods. The physical methods include techniques like laser ablation, lithography and high-energy irradiation, while chemical methods include techniques like chemical reduction, electrochemistry, and photochemical reduction. Physical and chemical methods of synthesis of nanoparticles involve expensive equipments and the use of toxic chemicals like sodium borohydride and N,N dimethylformamide which produce hazardous effects on health and environment. Presence of these toxic chemicals on synthesized nanoparticles has prevented their use in health care sector and biomedical applications. As a result, there is currently widespread interest in developing safe, biologically compatible, and environment-friendly methods to synthesize nanoparticles.

Biological Synthesis of Nanoparticles

Biological synthesis of nanoparticles is based on green chemistry approach that make use of unicellular and multicellular biological entities like plants, bacteria, fungus, viruses, actinomycetes, and yeast (Fig.1.). Synthesizing nanoparticles through biological entities as biological factories offers a safe, non-toxic and environment-friendly method of synthesizing nanoparticles with a wide range of sizes, shapes, compositions, and physicochemical properties. Generally, biological entities with a potential to accumulate heavy metals are suited for nanoparticle synthesis. Both, microorganisms and plants have the ability to uptake and accumulate inorganic metallic ions from polluted environment. The inherent ability of a biological entity to transform inorganic metal ions into metal nanoparticles intracellularly and extracellularly is the major advantage of biological synthesis. Organisms used in nanoparticle formation vary widely, from simple prokaryotic bacterial cells to complex eukaryotes. In natural systems, trace elements (heavy metals and metalloids) are important environmental pollutants, and are toxic even at very low concentrations. Microorganisms with a certain success have been used in metal bioremediation of contaminated subsurface environments. Plants have also shown great potential in heavy metal accumulation and detoxification.

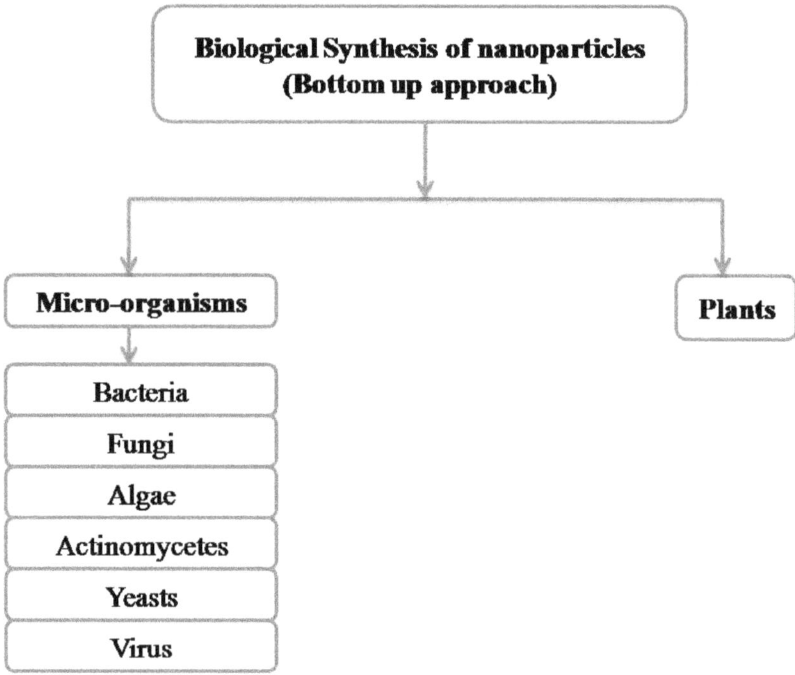

Fig. 1: List of living entities utilized for biological synthesis of nanoparticles.

Each biological entity has varying degree of biochemical processing capabilities that can be effectively used to synthesize particular metal or metal oxide nanoparticles. Biological synthesis of gold, silver, gold–silver alloy, selenium, tellurium, platinum, palladium, silica, titania, zirconia, quantum dots, magnetite and uraninite nanoparticles through biological synthesis have been reported. Furthermore, biosynthesis of metal nanoparticles is an environmentally friendly method without the use of toxic chemicals and expensive instrumental set-up in specific environmental condition.

Synthesis of Nanoparticles using Plants

The use of plants in recovery of noble metals from ore mines and runoffs is known as phytomining. It is a cost-effective, environmental-friendly method of synthesis compared to conventional methods. The natural phenomenon of heavy metal tolerance of plants has interested researchers to investigate the biological mechanisms of metal tolerance in hyperaccumulator plants. Gardea– Torresdey and his team in 2002 were the first to report on formation of gold and silver nanoparticles inside living plant, alfalfa by metal ion uptake from solid media. This study suggested that silver atoms accumulated inside the alfalfa plant tissues undergo nucleation and subsequently form nanoparticles.

The ability of plant extracts to reduce metal ions has been known since 1900s, although the nature of the reducing agents involved was not known. Reducing metal salts to nanoparticles with use of plants or plant part extracts have started to get significant importance only during the past two decades. Plant extracts may act both as reducing agents and stabilizing agents in the synthesis of nanoparticles. The source of the plant extract is known to influence the characteristics of the synthesized nanoparticles. Different plant extracts contain different concentrations and combinations of organic reducing agents. Most plants contain primary and secondary metabolites like enzymes, proteins, amino acids, vitamins, polysaccharides, and organic acids (citrates), reducing sugar, phenolic compounds, alkaloids, and terpenoids. Hydroxyl and carboxylic groups present in plant biomolecules may act as reducing agent and stabilizing agents in synthesis of metal nanoparticles. The stability of nanoparticles can be attributed to formation of stable bond between metallic nanoparticles and the phytochemicals present in the plant extract. Plant extracts can be used to reduce metal ions to nanoparticles in a single-step process (Fig. 2). Plant extract-mediated bioreduction involves mixing of the aqueous plant extract with an aqueous solution of the precursor metal salt. The reaction occurs at room temperature and will usually complete within few minutes to few hours. The nature of the plant extract, its concentration, concentration of the metal salt, pH, temperature and reaction time are known to affect the yield and physico-chemical characteristics of the synthesized nanoparticles.

Table 1. List of plants and its parts from which metals nanoparticles are synthesized

Name of the plant	Parts used	Nanoparticle Synthesized	Shape
Neem (*Azadirachta indica*)	Leaves	Silver	Spherical
Indian mallow (*Abutilon indicum*)	Leaves	Silver	Spherical
Parthenium (*Parthenium hysterophorus*)	Leaves	Silver	Irregular
Tulsi (*Ocimum sanctum*)	Roots	Silver	Spherical
Banana (*Musa paradisiaca*)	Peel	Cadmium sulfide	Nanoclusters

Green tea (*Camellia sinensis*)	Leaves	Gold	Spherical, Triangular, Irregular
Persimmon (*Diospyros kaki*)	Fruits	Bimetallic gold/ silver	Cubic
Henna (*Lawsonia inermis*)	Leaves	Iron	Hexagonal
Cape jasmine (*Gardenia jasminoides*)	Leaves	Iron	Rock like appearance
Periwinkle (*Catharanthu sroseus*)	Leaves	Palladium	Spherical
Alfalfa (*Medicago sativa*)	Leaves	Titanium-nickle alloy	Spherical

Plant based biosynthesis is relatively a straight forward process that can be easily scaled up for large-scale production of nanoparticles. Silver (Ag) and gold (Au) nanoparticles have been the focus of plant-based synthesis. Also, synthesis of iron, copper, platinum and palladium nanoparticles have been reported using plant extracts from diverse range of plant species.

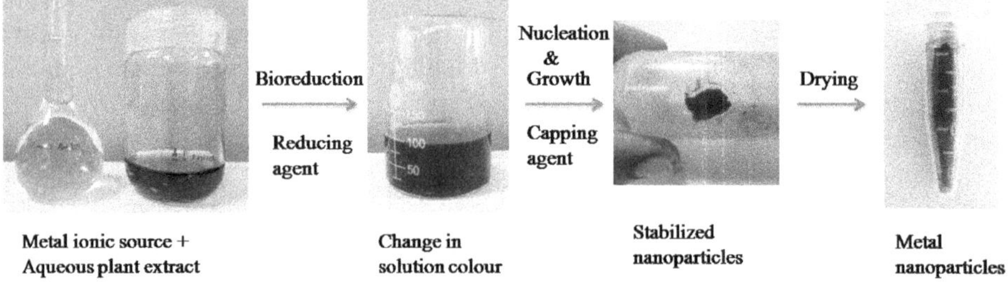

Fig. 2: Steps involved in biological synthesis of silver nanoparticles using dried leaf extract of *Andrographis paniculata* (Photo: Haripriya Shanmugam).

Microbial synthesis of metal nanoparticles

Microbial synthesis is also environment-friendly and compatible method for synthesis of nanoparticle, but culturing of microorganisms is expensive than plant extracts. Ability of microorganisms to actively interact with the metal contaminated environment arises from the composition of lipid-based amphipathic membranes. The bacterial membrane enables a variety of oxidation-reduction mechanisms to occur and to promote biochemical conversions. Microbes are able to produce inorganic nanoparticles either intracellularly or extracellularly according to the location where nanoparticles are formed (Table 2.).Microbial resistance to most toxic heavy metals are due to their chemical detoxification and energy-dependent ion efflux from the cell by membrane proteins that function either as ATPase or as chemiosmotic cation or proton anti-transporters. Therefore, microbes can detoxify metal ions either by reduction and/or precipitation of soluble toxic inorganic ions to insoluble non-toxic metal nanoclusters (Table 3.). Mechanism of metal nanoparticles synthesized by specific microorganisms is mentioned briefly in the forthcoming sections.

Table 2. Major difference between intracellular and extracellular synthesis of metal nanoparticles by microorganisms

Intracellular synthesis	Extracellular synthesis
Involves transporting metal ions into the microbial cell in the presence of enzymes	Involves trapping of metal ions on the surface of the cells and reducing metal ions in the presence of enzymes
Microorganisms are digested to collect nanoparticles	Nanoparticles are collected from the microbe culturing media.

Table 3. Types of microorganism involved in synthesis of metal nanoparticles

Type of micro-organism with localization	Microorganism	Metal nanoparticle synthesized	Shape
Bacteria-intracellular	*Bacillus subtilis*	Au	Octahedral inside cell wall
	Bacillus sp.	Ag	Periplasmic space
	Lactobacillus sp.	Au, Ag, Au–Ag	Hexagonal/Contour
	Escherichia coli	CdS	Spherical, elliptical
Bacteria-extracellular	Thermophilic bacteria	Magnetite	Octahedral
	Actinobacter sp.	Magnetite	Quasi-spherical
	Klebsiella aerogenes	CdS	Spherical on cell wall
	Rhodobacter sphaeroides	PbS	Spherical
Fungi-intracellular	Verticillium sp.	Ag	Cell wall, cytoplasmic membrane/ spherical
	Aspergillus flavus	Ag	Cell wall
Fungi- extracellular	*Trichoderma viride*	Ag	Spherical, rod-like
	Fusarium oxysporum	CdSe	Spherical
Actinomycetes-intracellular	*Rhodococcus* sp.	Au	Cell wall, cytoplasmic membrane
	Streptomyces sp.	Ag	Spherical
Actinomycetes-Extracellular	*Thermomonospora* sp.	Au	Spherical
Yeast-intracellular	*Saccharomyces cerevisiae*	Sb_2O_3	Spherical
	Candida glubrata	CdS	Spherical
Yeast-extracellular	Yeast strain MKY3	Ag	Hexagonal
Viruses - extracellular	Tobacco mosaic virus (TMV)	SiO_2, CdS, PbS and Fe_2O_3	Nanotubes on surface
Viruses - intracellular	Bacteriophage	ZnS, CdS	Quantum dot nanowires

*(**Source:** Narayanan and Sakthivel (2010) from Advances in Colloid and Interface Science)*

Bacteria

Bacteria can detoxify metal toxicity either by extracellular biomineralization, biosorption, complexation/precipitation or intracellular bioaccumulation. Extracellular synthesis of metal nanoparticles have more commercial applications in various fields. Bacteria can synthesis nanoparticles through chemolithotropic growth, use of metal ions for specific function (synthesis of magnetosomes) or terminal electron acceptors and detoxification mechanisms. Since metal ions have a positive charge and the bacterial cell wall, a negative charge (carboxylate groups) metal-ions accumulate in the diffusive part of the electrical double layer. It can easily be deposited into the cell surface matrix through electrostatic interaction at the molecular level by simple ionic binding or by bridging polymeric structures.

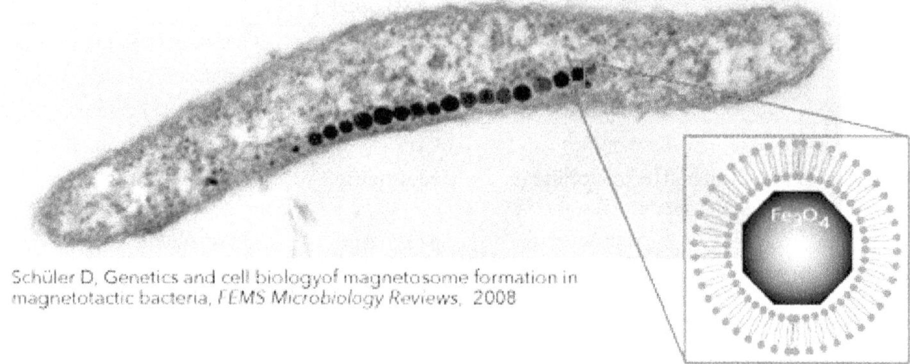

Fig. 3: Magnetosomes synthesized by magnetotactic bacteria

Richard Blakemore (1975) discovered magnetotactic bacteria (*Magnetospirillium magneticum*) that produce magnetosomes (magnetic nanoparticles) within the cell organelles (Fig 3.). Magnetosomes are membrane bound nanocrystals of magnetic iron minerals that help the bacteria to orient and swim along the Earth's geomagnetic and external field lines. This behavior of bacteria is known as magnetotaxis. Formation of magnetosomes in magnetotactic bacteria is a fascinating example for a highly controlled biomineralization process. Currently, magnetosomes are used in manufacture of magnetic tapes and printing inks, targeted drug delivery, cell separation and as contrast enhancement agents in magnetic resonance imaging.

Pseudomonas stutzeri, isolated from silver mines formed silver nanocrystals embedded in the organic matrix of the bacteria was the first report on the biosynthesis of silver nanoparticles. The bioreduction was initiated by electron transfer from NADH by NADH-dependent reductase. For metal nanoparticle synthesis, it is essential for bacteria to overcome toxicity of metals by binding them with various functional groups and proteins. Different metal binding proteins are secreted by bacteria. Apart from metal binding proteins, cyanobacterial polysaccharides have many uronic acid subunits, wherein carboxylic groups binds with the metals. Once inside the cell, the metals can be reduced through intrinsic metabolic process.

Fungi

Fungi have been frequently reported for their biosynthetic ability to synthesize both gold and silver nanoparticles. Fungi possess some additional attributes when compared to bacteria i.e., fungi secrete large amounts of proteins and enzymes per unit of biomass resulting in an increased quantity of nanoparticles formating. The nanoparticles formed inside the organism are usually smaller than extracellularly reduced nanoparticles. The size limit could be related to the particles nucleating inside the organisms. When the fungus mycelium is exposed to metal salt solution, osmotic stress is created and consequently produces enzymes/metabolites as defense mechanism. These extracellular enzyme and metabolites of the fungus catalyzes reduction of toxic metal ions to the non-toxic metal nanoparticles. Besides extracellular enzymes, bioactives like naphthoquinones and anthraquinones act as electron shuttle in metal reductions.

The plant pathogenic fungal strain *Fusarium oxysporum* is the most widely studied fungi towards synthesis of metal nanoparticles. The NADPH-dependent nitrate reductase enzyme purified from the fungus, *Fusarium oxysporium* have been used for the synthesis of gold and silver nanoparticles. In this case, enzymes transfer electrons through cytochromes to reduce metal ions. Once synthesized, the nanoparticles are stabilized by different proteins as capping agents. *Fusarium oxysporum* can also synthesize metal nanoparticles extracellularly by secretion of high amount of proteins and/or enzymes resulting in formation of highly stable gold and silver nanoparticles. Purified rhamanolipids from *Pseudomonas aeruginosa* were also used to synthesize silver nanoparticles.

Viruses

Viruses are considered as natural nanoparticles and its structure is considered as a nanocontainer. An attractive feature of viruses are the capsid proteins (dense surface covering) that form a highly reactive surface capable of interacting with metal ions. Tobacco mosaic virus (TMV) is a typical plant virus with approximately 2130 capsid protein molecules covering its surface. This array of proteins acts as attachment points for deposition of metals. Low concentrations of TMV's added to gold or silver salt precursors followed by adding plant extracts of *Nicotiana benthamiana* (Round-leaved native tobacco) or *Hordeum vulgare* (Barley) decreased the size and increased the number of nanoparticles synthesized. In this case, viral capsid could have involved in reduction of gold tetrachloride ion ($AuCl_4^-$) to gold ion (Au^+) to gold atom (Au^0) and formation of gold (Au) nanoparticles through electron transfer from tyrosine residues present on the surface. Viral capsid can also act as a template for symmetry directed synthesis of gold atom (Au^0) nanoparticles from a non-reducible gold precursor. Viruses are relatively less explored for synthesis of nanoparticles and extensive research is needed on scaling up process.

Yeasts

Yeasts are considered to be beneficial over bacteria for synthesis of metal nanoparticles, yeast can be easily controlled under laboratory circumstances, secretes large amount of enzymes and grows faster with simple nutrients. Yeast cells use a variety of detoxification mechanisms that cause chelation, bio-precipitation, biosorption and extracellular sequestration to overcome metal toxicity. *Candida glabrata* exposed to cadmium salts resulted in intracellular synthesis of cadmium sulfide (CdS) quantum dots. Likewise, silver nanoparticles were extracellularly synthesized by *Aspergillus fumigatus.*

Actinomycetes

Actinomycetes are well known for their antimicrobial activities and for synthesis of metal nanoparticles. Reduction of metal ions in actinomycetes is a result of interacting enzymes being released from its cell membrane and cell wall, while capping proteins stabilizes the formed nanoparticles. With actinomycetes, extracellular synthesis is the common pathway for synthesizing metal nanoparticles. Extracellular synthesis of silver nanoparticles using *Streptomyces* sp. and silver nitrate salt is due to nitrate reductase enzyme, responsible for bioreduction of nitrate to nitrite. Intracellular reduction of metal gold ions by the *Rhodococcus* sp. took place on the cell wall and cytoplasmic spaces.

Algae

Algae are eukaryotic photoautotrophs found in freshwater, salt water, or marshy wetlands and only a few of them are capable of accumulating heavy metals. Extract from unicellular alga, *Chlorella vulgari,* known for its high reproduction rate was found to produce gold nanoparticles at room temperature. The reason being, its cell contains twenty proteinogenic amino acids and proteins are primarily involved in reduction as well as size and shape control. So, proteins in the algal extract act as both reducing and stabilizing agent. Also, Marine alga, *Sargassum wightii* was capable of extracellular synthesis of gold, silver and gold/silver bimetallic nanoparticles. Likewise, edible blue-green alga (*Spirulina platensis*) in dried form was used for extracellular synthesis of gold, silver and gold/silver (Au/Ag) bimetallic nanoparticles. However, there are very few reports about biological synthesis of metal nanoparticles using algae.

Applications of Biologically Synthesized Metal Nanoparticles

- Gold nanoparticles are a promising scaffold for drug and gene delivery. It can be also used for hyperthermia cancer treatment.
- Silver nanoparticles have been widely used as antibacterial, antifungal, antiviral and anti-inflammatory agent. They are commercially utilized in wound dressings (bandages), pharmaceutical preparations, and medical implant coatings.

- Platinum and palladium nanoparticles are utilized in catalysis and electro-catalysis applications, chemical sensors, optoelectronics, and anti-bacterial activity applications.
- Non-noble metallic nanoparticles like iron, copper, zinc oxide, and selenium have been used in cosmetic formulations and anti-bacterial activity applications.
- Gold–silver alloy nanoparticles biosynthesized by yeast cells were used to fabricate electrochemical vanillin sensor towards determination of vanillin content in the vanilla beans.

Biologically synthesized nanoparticles have been used in a variety of applications as drug carriers for targeted delivery, cancer treatment, gene therapy, antibacterial agents, biosensors, catalysts, separation science, and magnetic resonance imaging. Gold and silver nanoparticles are the most commonly synthesized, but silver nanoparticles are widely utilized in consumer products. At present, biosynthesis of nanomaterials are confined to metals, some metal sulfides, and very few metal oxides. Majority of metals are toxic to most microorganisms, especially silver ions. A shift in biological synthesis of nanoparticles from bacteria to fungi and plants was noticed in the recent past. Although biological methods are regarded as safe, cost-effective and environmental friendly method, important challenge relies on scaling up the production of nanoparticles. It includes limitations like culturing of microbes, chances of mutation and biomass harvesting, which is time-consuming and having difficulty in control over particle size, shape and crystallinity. Despite its limitation, research and product development with biologically synthesized nanoparticles fascinate people around the world.

Suggested Reading Materials

- Synthesis of Nanoparticles and Nanomaterials: Biological Approaches 2017. Zhypargul Abdullaeva © Springer International Publishing AG.
- Green Synthesis of Metallic Nanoparticles via Biological Entities. 2015. Monaliben Shah , Derek Fawcett , Shashi Sharma , Suraj Kumar Tripathy and Gerrard Eddy Jai Poinern. Materials, 8, 7278–7308.
- Green synthesis of metal nanoparticles using plants. 2011. Siavash Iravani. Green Chemistry,13, 2638-2650.
- Biosynthesis of Nanoparticles by Microorganisms and Their Applications. 2011. Xiangqian Li, Huizhong Xu, Zhe-Sheng Chen, and Guofang Chen. Journal of Nanomaterials. doi:10.1155/2011/270974.

Self-assessment Questions

1. First report on formation of silver nanoparticles inside the living plants is from

   a. Neem b. Parthenium

   c. Alfalfa d. Persimmon

2. Most commonly used metal nanoparticles in consumer products is

   a. Gold   b. Silver

   c. Platinum   d. Copper

3. ____________________act as reducing agent in synthesis of metal nanoparticles from plants.

4. ____________________acts as capping agents in synthesis of metal nanoparticles from microbes.

5. Biologically synthesized ______________ nanoparticles are used in hyperthermia cancer treatment.

6. Synthesis of metal nanoparticles through fungi is advantageous over bacteria. **True/False**

7. Synthesis of nanoparticles through biological methods is eco-friendly. **True/False**

8. List the drawbacks in conventional method of synthesis of nanoparticles?

9. Difference between intracellular and extracellular synthesis of metal nanoparticles from microorganisms?

10. What are magnetosomes?

11. Applications of biologically synthesized metal nanoparticles?

12. How synthesis of metal nanoparticle using plants and microorganisms vary?

13. Write a brief note on mechanism of nanoparticle synthesis by bacteria?

14. Explain biological synthesis of nanoparticle using plants with a schematic diagram?

15. Write in detail on biological synthesis of nanoparticles using plants and microorganism?

7

Particle Size Analyzer: Principle, Components and Applications

Dr K. Raja and Dr. S.Marimuthu

The particle is defined as the discrete sub-portion of a substance. The most common types of materials consisting of particles are powders and granules, suspensions, emulsions and slurries , aerosols and sprays. The particle size is a valuable indicator of quality and performance of particulate materials. Measuring particle size and understanding how it affects the products and processes can be critical to the success of many manufacturing businesses. Size and shape impact the compaction properties of materials where smaller particles dissolve more quickly in a dispersion media which leads to higher suspension viscosities than larger ones. Smaller droplet size and higher surface charge (zeta potential) will typically improve suspension and emulsion stability. The Powder or droplets in the range of 2-5μm aerosolize better and will penetrate into lungs deeper than larger sizes.

The significance of zeta potential is that its value can be related to the stability of colloidal dispersions. The zeta potential indicates the degree of repulsion between adjacent, similarly charged particles in dispersion. For molecules and particles that are small enough, a high zeta potential will confer stability, i.e., the solution or dispersion will resist aggregation. When the potential is low, attraction exceeds repulsion and the dispersion will break and flocculate. Hence, it is important to measure and control the particle size distribution and zeta potential of many products. The particle size analyzer is a user-friendly system for colloidal, nanoparticles and macromolecules characterization. It can determine particle size distribution, particle zeta potential (related to the magnitude of the electrical charge at the particle surface) and molecular weight of large substances dispersed in water

Particle Size Measurement

Particle size is the most important physical property of particulate samples and as a critical parameter which decides the fate of many products. It directly influences the material properties *viz.*, reactivity or dissolution rate, stability in suspension, efficacy of delivery, texture and feel, appearance, flow ability and handling, viscosity, packing density and porosity

Defining particle size: Particles are three dimensional objects, and unless they are perfect spheres (e.g. emulsions or bubbles), they cannot be fully described by a single dimension such as a radius or diameter. In order to simplify the measurement process, it is often convenient to define the particle size using the concept of equivalent spheres. In this case the particle size is defined by the diameter of an equivalent sphere having the same property as the actual particle such as volume or mass for example. It is important to realize that different measurement techniques use different equivalent sphere models and therefore will not necessarily give exactly the same result for the particle diameter.

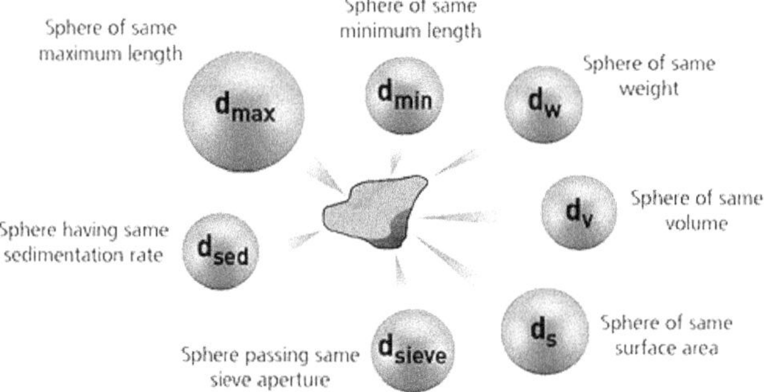

Courtesy: Malvern Instruments

Fig. 1: Concept of equivalent sphere

The equivalent sphere concept works very well for regular shaped particles. But in the case of irregular shaped particles it may not always be appropriate for irregular shaped particles, such as needles or plates, where the size in at least one dimension can differ significantly from that of the other dimensions

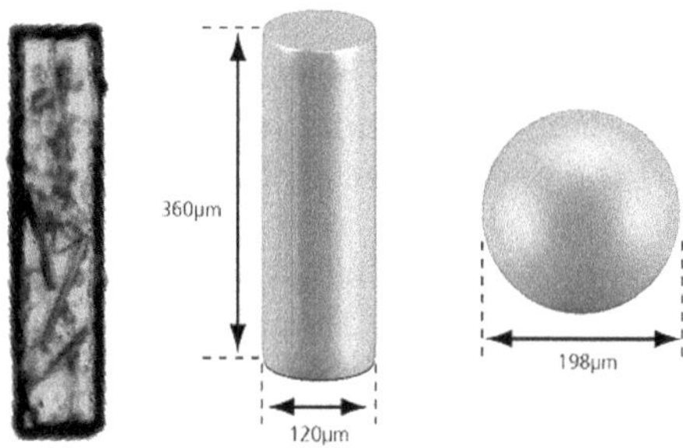

Courtesy: Malvern Instruments

Fig. 2: Volume equivalent rod and sphere of a needle shaped particle

In the case of the rod shaped particle shown in the image above, a volume equivalent sphere would give a particle diameter of 198µm, which is not a very accurate description of its true dimensions. However, we can also define the particle as a cylinder with the same volume which has a length of 360µm and a width of 120µm. This approach more accurately describes the size of the particle and may provide a better understanding of the behavior of this particle during processing or handling for example. Many particle sizing techniques are based on a simple 1-dimensional sphere equivalent measuring concept, and this is often perfectly adequate for the required application. Measuring particle size in two or more dimensions can sometimes be desirable but can also present some significant measurement and data analysis challenges. Therefore careful consideration is advisable when choosing the most appropriate particle sizing technique for your application.

Particle Size Distributions

Unless the sample to be characterized is perfectly mono disperse, i.e. every single particle has exactly the same dimensions, it will consist of a statistical distribution of particles of different sizes. It is common practice to represent this distribution in the form of either a frequency distribution curve, or a cumulative (undersize) distribution curve.

Weighted distributions: A particle size distribution can be represented in different ways with respect to the weighting of individual particles. The weighting mechanism will depend upon the measuring principle being used.

Number weighted distributions: A counting technique such as image analysis will give a number weighted distribution where each particle is given equal weighting irrespective of its size. This is most often useful where knowing the absolute number of particles is important - in foreign particle detection for example - or where high resolution (particle by particle) is required.

Volume weighted distributions: Static light scattering techniques such as laser diffraction will give a volume weighted distribution. Here the contribution of each particle in the distribution

relates to the volume of that particle (equivalent to mass if the density is uniform), i.e. the relative contribution will be proportional to size. This is often extremely useful from a commercial perspective as the distribution represents the composition of the sample in terms of its volume/mass.

Intensity weighted distributions: Dynamic light scattering techniques will give an intensity weighted distribution, where the contribution of each particle in the distribution relates to the intensity of light scattered by the particle. For example, using the Rayleigh approximation, the relative contribution for very small particles will be proportional to size.

When comparing particle size data for the same sample measured by different techniques, it is important to realize that the types of distribution being measured and reported can produce very different particle size results. This is clearly illustrated in the example below, for a sample consisting of equal numbers of particles with diameters of 5nm and 50nm. The number weighted distribution gives equal weighting to both types of particles, emphasising the presence of the finer 5 nm particles, whereas the intensity weighted distribution has a signal one million times higher for the coarser 50nm particles. The volume weighted distribution is intermediate between the two (Fig.3).

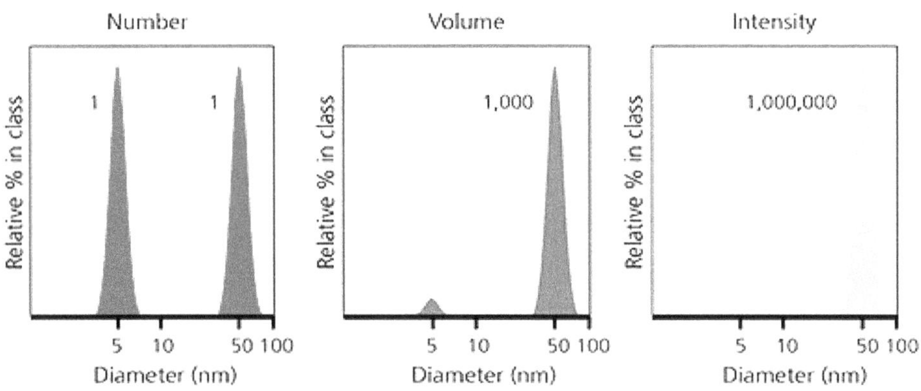

Courtesy: Malvern Instruments

Fig. 3: Example of number, volume and intensity weighted particle size distributions for the same sample

Particle Size Measurement Techniques

There are wide ranges of particle size characterization techniques such as laser diffraction analysis; dynamic light scattering techniques and image analyzing are available. Each technique has it relative strength and limitations. In this chapter the principle, components and application of dynamic light scattering technique is described for measuring the particle size and distribution of sample

Dynamic Light Scattering

Dynamic light scattering (DLS) is also referred to as Photon Correlation Spectroscopy (PCS) or Quasi-Elastic Light Scattering (QELS). This technique is well established, eco-friendly and non-invasive one, which could measure the size of particle in the range of 0 .001 – 6 microns.

Principle

Dynamic light scattering uses Brownian motion and relates this phenomenon with size of the particles. Microscopic particles exhibit random motion while they are dispersed in a solvent due to thermal motion; Small particles are pushed in random motion due to the bombardment of solvent molecules that encircle them. Hence, smaller particles move faster and travel longer distances, while larger particles move slower and travel shorter distances. The larger the particle, the slower will be the Brownian motion. When particles under movement in the liquid medium are illuminated with a laser, the intensity of the scattered light fluctuates over very short timescales at a rate that is dependent upon the size of the particles; smaller particles are displaced further by the solvent molecules and move more rapidly. Analysis of these intensity fluctuations yields the velocity of the Brownian motion and hence the particle size using the Stokes-Einstein relationship (explained elsewhere in this chapter). The diameter measured in this technique is called the hydrodynamic diameter and refers to the way a particle diffuses within a fluid. The diameter obtained by this technique is that of a sphere that has the same translational diffusion coefficient as the particle being measured.

The temperature of the medium needs to be stable for normal Brownian motion of particles, otherwise convection currents in the sample will cause non-random movements of particles. Similarly liquid viscosity also affects the motion of particles, since it is related the temperature. Higher temperatures or lower fluid viscosity will result in a higher frequency vibration

When light strikes moving or "vibrating" particles in the liquid medium, the frequency of the light exhibits a Doppler shift. The frequency is shifted when reflected off a moving surface (of the particle). It increases when the particle is moving towards the incident light and decreases when the particle is moving away. If a laser beam illuminates a cuvette containing particles dispersed in a liquid medium, and the speckle is focused on the screen and freezed for a moment, the similar speckle pattern will be obtained as show in the Fig. 4. The dark and bright spots are appeared in the speckle, where dark spaces are due to the phase additions of the scattered light are mutually destructive and nullify each other. The bright spots in the speckle pattern are where the light scattered from the particles arrives with the same phase and interfere constructively to form a bright patch. The particles are under constant motion in Brownian movement and hence a speckle pattern is also changing accordingly, and forming new patterns. The rate of intensity fluctuations between the two phases of interferences depends on the size of the particles. The small particles cause the intensity to fluctuate more rapidly than the large ones.

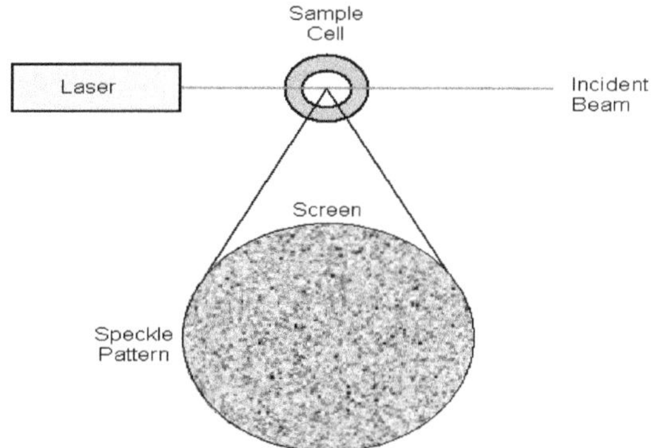

Courtesy: Malvern Instruments

Fig. 4: Illustration of speckle pattern of medium illuminated with laser light

Stokes Einstein law: Relating Particle Size to Particle Motion: The rate of movement of particles in a liquid medium is related to the translational diffusion coefficient D, which is calculated by Stoke's and Einstein's equation:

$$D = kT / 3\pi\eta Dv$$

Where

D is the diffusion coefficient

k is the Boltzmann's constant

η is the solvent viscosity

T is the temperature

Dv is the particle diameter

Working Principle

Capturing intensity fluctuations due to Brownian motion and converting them directly for particle size calculation are difficult and hence auto correlator is used to relate intensity fluctuations to assess the particle size. Normally, a series of frequency-intensity distributions for a wide range of particle sizes are prepared in advance and the measured power spectrum is compared to calculate the particle size distribution of the particles in the sample.

A correlator is basically a signal comparator, designed to measure the degree of similarity between two signals, or one signal with itself at varying time intervals. If the intensity of a signal is compared between time intervals and the intensities of signals will not be the similar, and hence cannot be correlated. However, if the intensity of signal at time = t is compared to the intensity at very small time later (t+δt) as shown in Fig. 5, there will be a strong relationship or correlation between the two signals. Even, if the signal, at t is compared to the signal at t+2δt, there will be a reasonable comparison or correlation between the two signals, under random process such as Brownian motion, but the correlation will not be as good as the comparison between t and t+δt. The degree of correlation is reducing with time. If the signals at t+2δt, t+3δt, t+4δt etc. are compared with the signal at t, the correlation of Dynamic Light Scattering (DLS) principle can be used to determine the size distribution profile of small particles in suspension or polymers in solution. It can also be used to probe the behaviour of complex fluids such as concentrated polymer solutions.

a signal arriving from a random source will decrease with time until at some time, effectively $t = \infty$, there will be no correlation. The time at which the correlation starts to significantly decay is an indication of the mean size of the sample. The steeper the line indicates, the more monodisperse of the sample. Conversely, the more extended the decay becomes, the greater the sample polydispersity. The particles in dispersion are in a constant, random Brownian motion and cause the intensity of scattered light to fluctuate as a function of time. The correlator will construct the correlation function of the scattered intensity. Size is obtained from the correlation function by using various algorithms. Ex. Particle size and the distribution pattern of ZnO and TiO_2 nanoparticles synthesized by chemical method analyzed under dynamic light scattering method using 90º or 173º at 25ºC shows the average particle size of 80.2 and 131.8 nm (Fig.6)

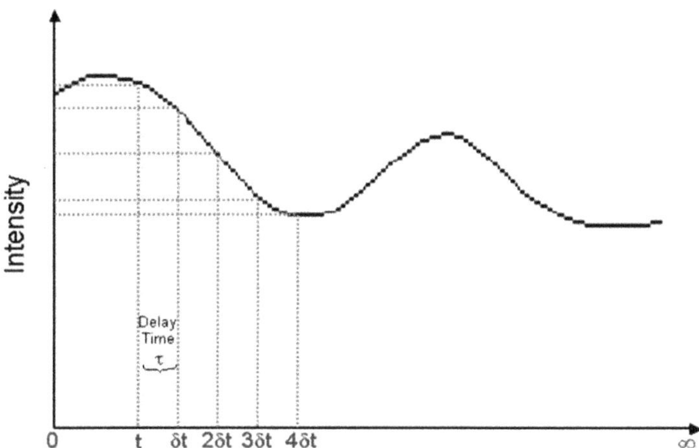

Courtesy: Malvern Instruments

Calculation Results

Peak No.	S.P.Area Ratio	Mean	S. D.	Mode
1	1.00	81.6 nm	5.6 nm	80.2 nm
2	---	--- nm	--- nm	--- nm
3	---	--- nm	--- nm	--- nm
Total	---	81.6 nm	5.6 nm	80.2 nm

Cumulant Operations

Z-Average : 25834.8 nm

PI : 3.323

ZnO NPs

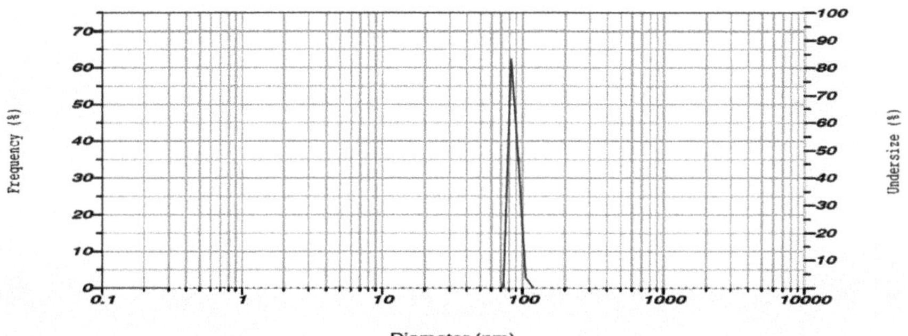

Fig. 5: Schematic illustration showing the fluctuation in the intensity of scattered light as a function of time

Calculation Results

Peak No.	S.P.Area Ratio	Mean	S. D.	Mode
1	1.00	134.8 nm	10.4 nm	131.8 nm
2	---	--- nm	--- nm	--- nm
3	---	--- nm	--- nm	--- nm
Total	---	134.8 nm	10.4 nm	131.8 nm

Cumulant Operations

Z-Average : 13265.0 nm

PI : 6.968

TiO_2 NPs

Frequency (%)

Undersize (%)

Diameter (nm)

Courtesy: Dileep Kumar, 2015

Fig. 6: Particle average size and intensity distribution of ZnO and TiO_2 nanoparticles

Components / Optical Setup of Dynamic Light Scattering:

The optical setup of dynamic light scattering is shown in Fig.7. The source laser light is produced from the laser light source which illuminates the particles of sample kept in the cuvette cell. As the light hits the particles, they scatter the light. The scattered light signal is collected with one of two detectors, either at a 90 degree (right angle) or 173 degree (back angle) scattering angle. The provision of both detectors allows more flexibility in choosing measurement conditions. Particles can be dispersed in a variety of liquids. Only liquid refractive index and viscosity needs to be known for interpreting the measurement results. The time acquisition for measuring the particle size is two or less than two minutes. DLS measures the particle size in the range of 0.3nm to 8 μm

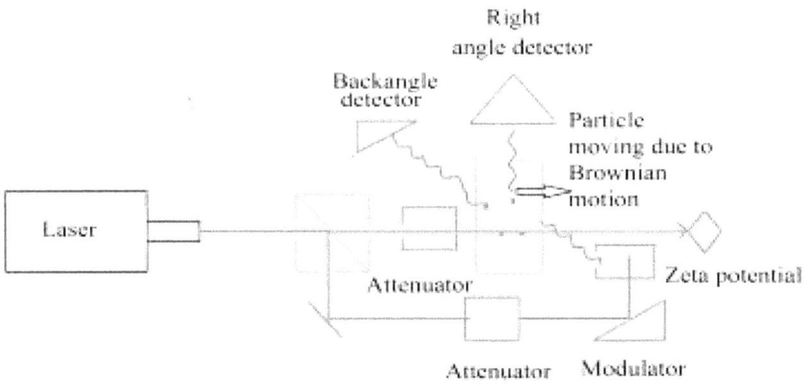

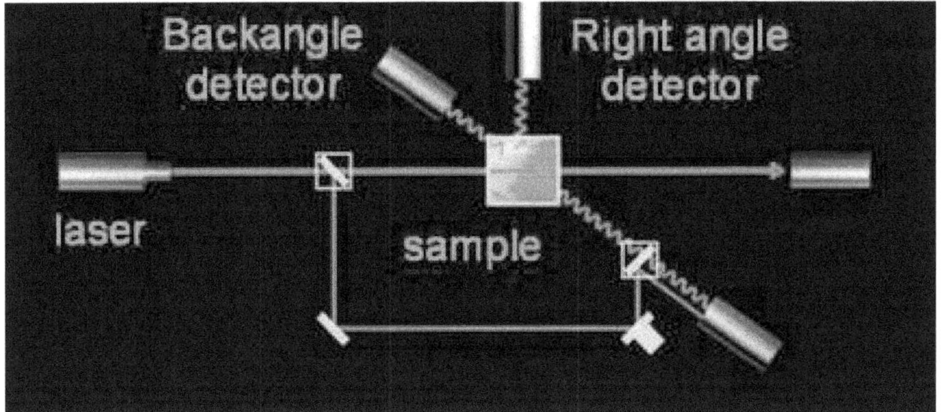

Courtesy: Horiba Instruments

Fig. 7: Optical setup for dynamic light scattering (DLS) nanoparticle size analyzer

Zeta Potential of Nanomaterials

The surface potential at electrical double layer at shear plane is called as zeta potential. Zeta potential depends on the interaction between particle and colloidal dispersion system, indicating particles' dispersion stability. This value of surface charge is useful for understanding and predicting interactions between particles in suspension. Manipulating zeta potential is a method of enhancing suspension stability for formulation work, or speeding particle flocculation in applications such as water treatment. The stability behaviour of the colloid particles are depicted in the below table

Zeta potential (mV)]	Stability behavior of the colloid
from 0 to ±5	Rapid coagulation or flocculation
from ±10 to ±30	Incipient instability
from ±30 to ±40	Moderate stability
from ±40 to ±60	Good stability
more than ±61	Excellent stability

An electrophoretic light scattering technique is used to calculate the Zeta potential, where an alternative potential to the solution is applied which induces oscillating movement in particles. The frequency of the scattered light by the particles is shifted during the oscillation compared to the fundamental beam due to Doppler Effect. Electric voltage charge of particles is obtained by detecting signal after oscillation with reference light interference, measuring frequency variation. Figure 8 exhibits the zeta potential of chemically synthesized nanoparticles and the polymer (CMC) based hormone (IAA) loaded nanoemulsion where the synthesized ZnO NPs shows the zeta potentials of 26.4 mV, and this reveals the stability and free from agglomeration of ZnO NPs. Similarly, CMC based IAA loaded nanoemulsion has the zeta potential of -36.3 mV which shows the stability of the emulsion since the zeta potential is above the range of -30 and + 30 mV. The zeta potential measured in the range of -200 mV to 200 mV with the data acquisition time of less than one minute. In the zeta analyzer, laser light is divided into two beams as input light and reference light. Scattered light by sample particles and reference light modulated by the modulator interfere in the prism are detected and the detected signals are changed into digital signal to calculate the zeta potential.

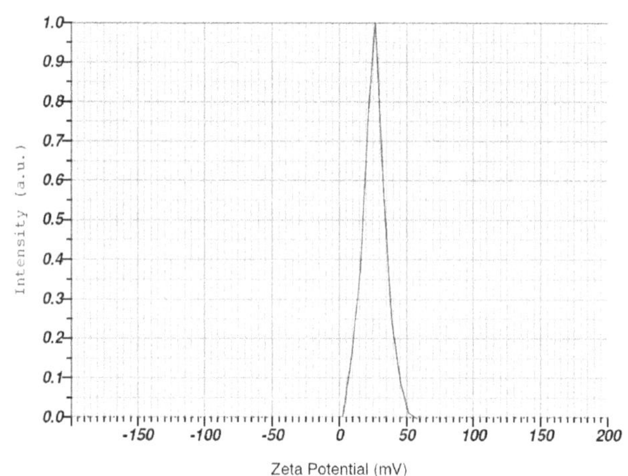

Courtesy: Sakthivel, 2016

Fig. 8: Zeta potential of ZnO NPs and Polymer based nanoemulsion

Applications

- Particle size analyzer is a non-destructive and eco-friendly method has wide application in the fields of cosmetics, ceramics, drug delivery, food and beverages, nanotechnology characterization, cement, nutraceuticals, pharmaceuticals aerosols, agriculture, pigments and inks, paper, polymer and plastics etc., In all theses area, the particle size analyzer analysis the particle size for describing the quality of product and zeta potential to address the stability of materials.
- DLS technique preliminary used for the size determination for standardizing the protocol to synthesize nanoparticles

Advantages

- It is a simple and faster technique for the determination of size and stability of the particulate materials
- It follows simple sample preparation
- Interpretation of results is simple and easy

- Simple instrumentation

Limitations

- It assumes all particles as spherical in shape
- Requires a special dispersant agents depending upon the nature of the particles
- It needs refractive index of both the dispersant and sample

Self-assessment Questions

1. Define zeta potential
2. Define Brownian motion
3. Principle of the Dynamic Light Scattering
4. What is the significance of autocorrelator
5. Describe the optical setup of dynamic light scattering system with illustration
6. Write the principle of zeta potential
7. How do you correlate the zeta potential with stability of colloid particles?
8. What are the factors affect the Brownian motion of particles in the liquid media?
9. List the merits and demerits of particle size analyzer
10. What is the significance of speckle pattern of light scattering?
11. List the field of applications of particle size analyzer

Fill in the blanks

1. Dynamic light scattering measure the zeta potential of particles in the range of _________ mV
2. DLS measures the size by assuming all particle as _______________ in shape
3. DLS measures the particle size in the range _________________________
4. Particles exhibit ______________ motion when dispersed in a solvent
5. The frequency of the light exhibits ________________effect when it strikes the particles vibrating in the liquid media
6. Nanoemulsion with – 60mVzeta potential exhibits _______________________ stability
7. Zeta potential measured using the techniques called _____________________
8. _________________ law is used to relate the particle size to particle motion

8

Scanning Electron Microscopy: Principle, Components and Applications

Dr. M. Kannan

Scanning Electron Microscope functions exactly as their optical counterparts except that they use a focused beam of electrons instead of light to "image" the specimen and gain information as to its structure and composition. Given sufficient light, the unaided human eye can distinguish two points 0.2 mm apart. If the points are closer together, they will appear as a single point. This distance is called the resolving power or resolution of the eye. Similarly, light microscopes use visible light (400- 700nm) and transparent lenses to see objects as small as about one micrometer (one millionth of a meter), such as a red blood cell (7 μm) or a human hair (100 μm). Light microscope has a magnification of about 1000x and enables the eye to resolve objects separated by 200 nm. Electron Microscopes were developed due to the limitations of light microscopes, which are limited by the physics of light. Electron Microscopes are capable of much higher magnifications and have a greater resolving power than a light microscope, allowing it to see much smaller objects at sub cellular, molecular and atomic level. The smallest the wavelength of the illuminating sources is the best resolution of the microscope.

De Broglie defined the **wavelength of** moving particles (**electron**) $\lambda = h/mv$, Where λ= wavelength of particles, h= Planck's constant, m= mass of the particle (electron), v= velocity of the particles; after substituting the known values, $\lambda = 12.3$ A°/V

The resolution of an optical microscope is defined as the shortest distance between two points on a specimen that can still be distinguished by the observer or camera system as separate entities. Resolution **(r)** = λ/ **(2NA)**, Where λ is the imaging wavelength, NA is objective numerical aperture.

Magnification is the process of enlarging the appearance, not physical size, of something. Magnification is defined as the ratio of image distance versus object distance

M= v/u, Where M= magnification, u= object distance, v= image distance

Magnification is also defined as the ratio of the resolving power of the eye to resolving power (δ) of the microscope M= δ eye/ δ microscope

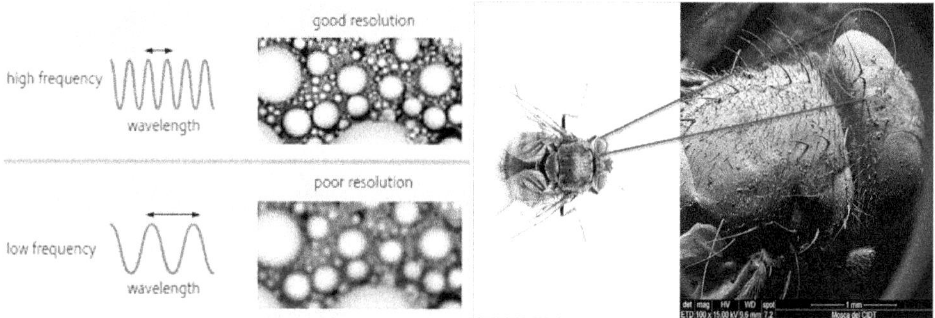

Resolution **Magnification**

Difference between light microscope and electron microscope

Sl. No.	Feature	Light microscope	Electron microscope
1.	Electromagnetic spectrum	Visible light, 400-700nm Colours visible	Electrons, app. 4nm Monochrome
2.	Maximum resolving power	app. 200nm	0.5nm with very fine detail
3.	Maximum magnification	x1000 to x1500	x500000
4.	Radiation source	Tungsten or quartz halogen lamp	High voltage (50kV) tungsten lamp, Lanthanum hexaboride
5.	Lenses	Glass	Electro magnetics
6.	Interior	Air-filled	Vacuum
7.	Focusing screen	Human eye (retina), photographic film	Fluorescent (TV) screen, Photographic film
8.	Preparation of specimens	Temporary mounts living or dead	Tissues must be dehydrated = dead
9.	Fixation	Alcohol	OsO_4 or $KMnO_4$
10.	Embedding medium	Wax	Resin
11.	Sectioning of specimen	Hand or microtome sectioning < 20µm slice Whole cells visible	Ultra microtome sectioning < 50nm slices Parts of cells visible
12.	Staining	Water soluble dyes	Heavy metals
13.	Support for sample	Glass slide	Copper grid

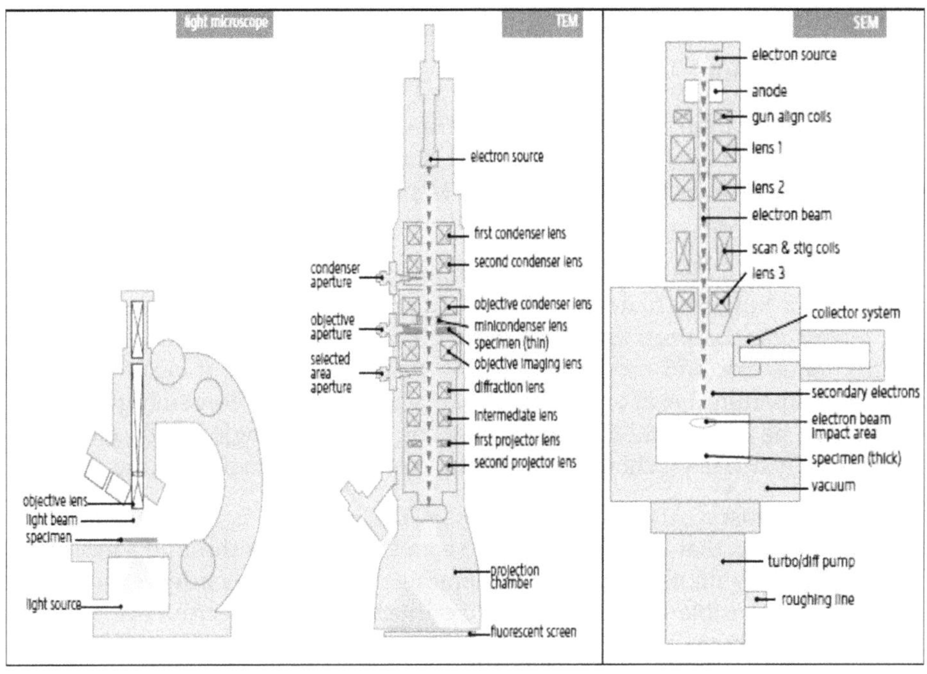

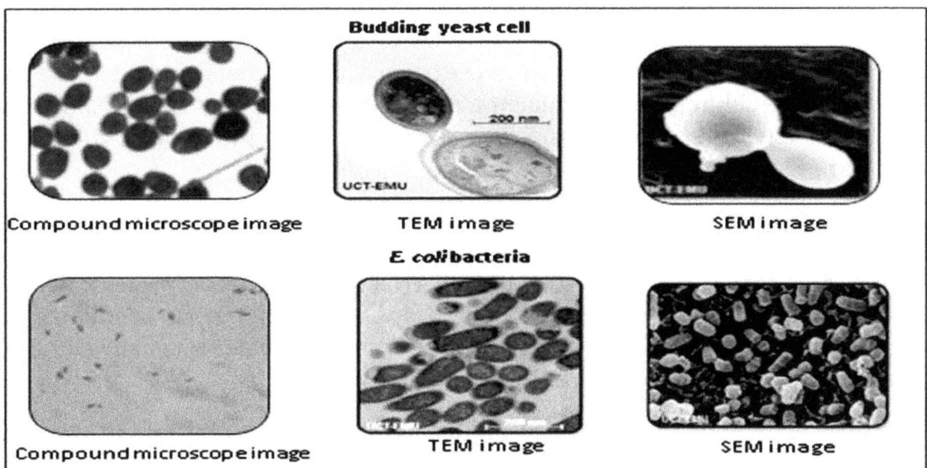

Working Principles of SEM

A beam of electrons is formed by the electron source and accelerated toward the specimen using a positive electrical potential. The electron beam is confined and focused using metal apertures and magnetic lenses into a thin, focused, monochromatic beam. Electrons in the beam interact with the atoms of the specimen, producing signals that contain information about its surface topography, composition and other electrical properties. These interactions and effects are detected and transformed into an image.

Components of SEM

Electron Column

The electron column is where the electron beam is generated under vacuum, focused to a small diameter, and scanned across the surface of a specimen by electromagnetic deflection coils. The lower portion of the column is called the specimen chamber.

Electron gun: An electron beam is thermionically emitted from an electron gun fitted with a tungsten filament cathode. Tungsten has the highest melting point and lowest vapour pressure of all metals, thereby allowing it to be heated for electron emission, and because of its low cost. Other types of electron emitters include lanthanum hexaboride (LaB_6) cathodes, and field emission guns (FEG), which may be of the cold-cathode type using tungsten single crystal emitters or the thermally assisted Schottky type, using emitters of zirconium oxide.

Condenser Lenses: After the beam passes the anode it is influenced by two condenser lenses that cause the beam to converge and pass through a focal point. In conjunction with the selected accelerating voltage the condenser lenses are primarily responsible for determining the intensity of the electron beam when it strikes the specimen.

Apertures: The function of these apertures is to reduce and exclude extraneous electrons in the lenses. The final lens aperture located below the scanning coils determines the diameter or spot size of the beam at the specimen. The spot size on the specimen will in part determine the resolution and depth of field. Decreasing the spot size will allow for an increase in resolution and depth of field with a loss of brightness.

Scanning System: Images are formed by rastering the electron beam across the specimen using deflection coils inside the objective lens. The stigmator or astigmatism corrector is located in the objective lens and uses a magnetic field in order to reduce aberrations of the electron beam. The electron beam should have a circular cross section when it strikes the specimen however it is usually elliptical thus the stigmator acts to control this problem.

Specimen Chamber: The lower portion of the column is specimen stage and controls are located. Specimens are mounted and secured onto the stage which is controlled by a goniometer. The secondary electrons from the specimen are attracted to the detector by a positive charge manual stage controls are found on the front side of the specimen chamber for x-y-z movement.

Electron Detectors: Detectors collect the signal generated from interaction of beam with specimen. Electronic detectors convert the signal into digital images and most often collected signal are secondary electrons by secondary electron detector (Everhart–Thornley) backscattered electrons by backscattered electrons detector (Solid-State detector) and X-rays signal by Energy Dispersive Spectrometer (EDS) detector.

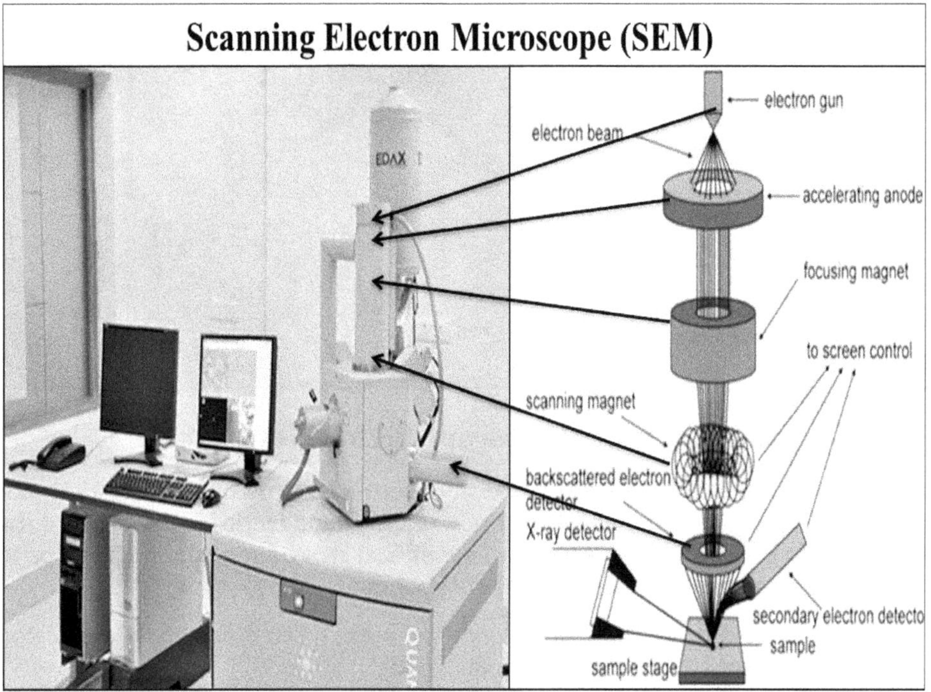

Vacuum System: Vacuum is produced by an oil diffusion pump backed by a mechanical pump. In the diffusion pump a stream of hot oil vapor strikes and pushes air molecules toward a mechanical pump that expels them from the system. A mechanical pump and valve system are used to preevacuate the system because a diffusion pump only operates after a vacuum is created. If the column is in a gas filled environment, electrons will be scattered collide with air molecules which would lead to reduction of the beam intensity and stability. Similarly, other gas molecules, which could come from the sample or the microscope itself, could form compounds and condense on the sample. This would lower the contrast and obscure detail in the image. The chemical and thermal stability is necessary for a well-functioning filament (gun pressure). The field emission gun, LaB_6 and tungsten filament requires ~ 10^{-10}, ~ 10^{-6} and 10^{-4} Torr, respectively. Hence, gun column of electron microscope require vacuum to facilitate the electrons signals from the sample to the detector for better imaging.

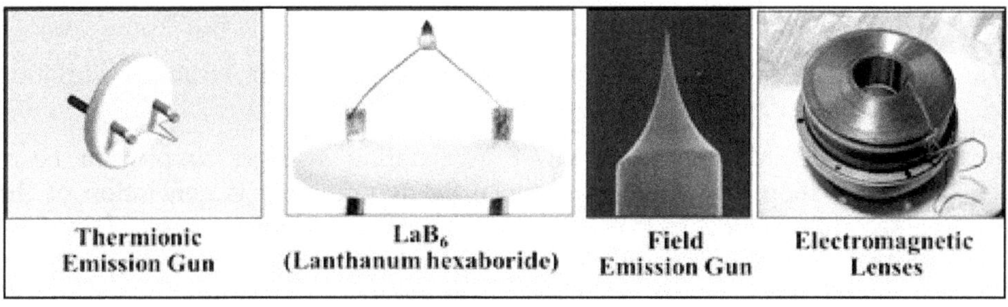

Detectors
X-rays: Energy dispersive spectrometer (EDS)
Secondary electron detector: (Everhart-Thornley)
Backscattered electron detector:(Solid-State Detector)

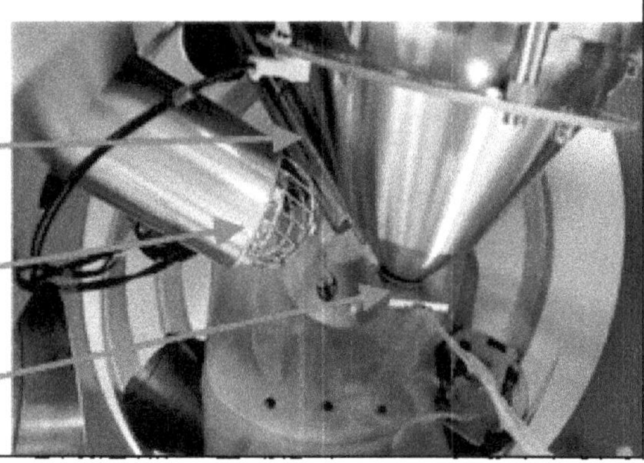

How Scanning Electron Microscope (SEM) Works

Ernst Ruska and Max Knoll developed first electron microscope during 1931with resolution of 100nm and later by addition of electromagnetic lenses, brought the resolution to 0.05nm. SEM is similar to the optical stereo-binocular microscope to observe the morphology and shape of the specimen.

- The electron gun produces an electron beam when tungsten wire is heated by current and accelerated by the anode.
- The beam travels in the vacuum column through electromagnetic fields and lenses, which focus the beam down toward the sample.
- A mechanism of deflection coils enables to guide the beam so that it scans the surface of the sample in a raster pattern.
- When the incident beam touches the surface of the sample and produces signals *viz.*,
  - Secondary electrons (SE)
  - Auger electrons
  - Back scattered electrons (BSE)
  - Characteristic X – Rays
  - Cathodoluminescence
- The emitted signals are trapped by electrical detectors, convert into digital images and displayed on a screen as digital image.
- Provides information sample's elemental composition, structural variation and morphology.
- In the SEM, use much lower accelerating voltages to prevent beam penetration into the sample since the requirement is generation of the secondary electrons from the true surface structure of a sample. Therefore, it is common to use low kV, in the range 1-5kV for biological samples, even though the SEMs are capable of up to 30 kV.

Interaction of Electron Beam with Specimen

When the primary electron beam interacts with the sample, the electrons lose energy by repeated random scattering and absorption within a teardrop-shaped volume of the specimen known as the interaction volume, which extends from less than 100 nm to approximately 10 μm into the surface. The size of the interaction volume depends on the electron's landing energy, the atomic number of the specimen and the specimen's density. The energy exchange between the electron beam and the sample results in the reflection of high-energy back scattered electrons by elastic scattering, emission of low energy secondary, auger electrons by inelastic scattering and the emission of electromagnetic radiation (X-rays and cathodoluminescence), each of which can be detected by respective detectors. The beam current absorbed by the specimen can also be detected and used to create images of the distribution of specimen current. Electronic amplifiers of various types are used to amplify the signals, electronic detectors convert the signals into digital images and displayed on a computer monitor.

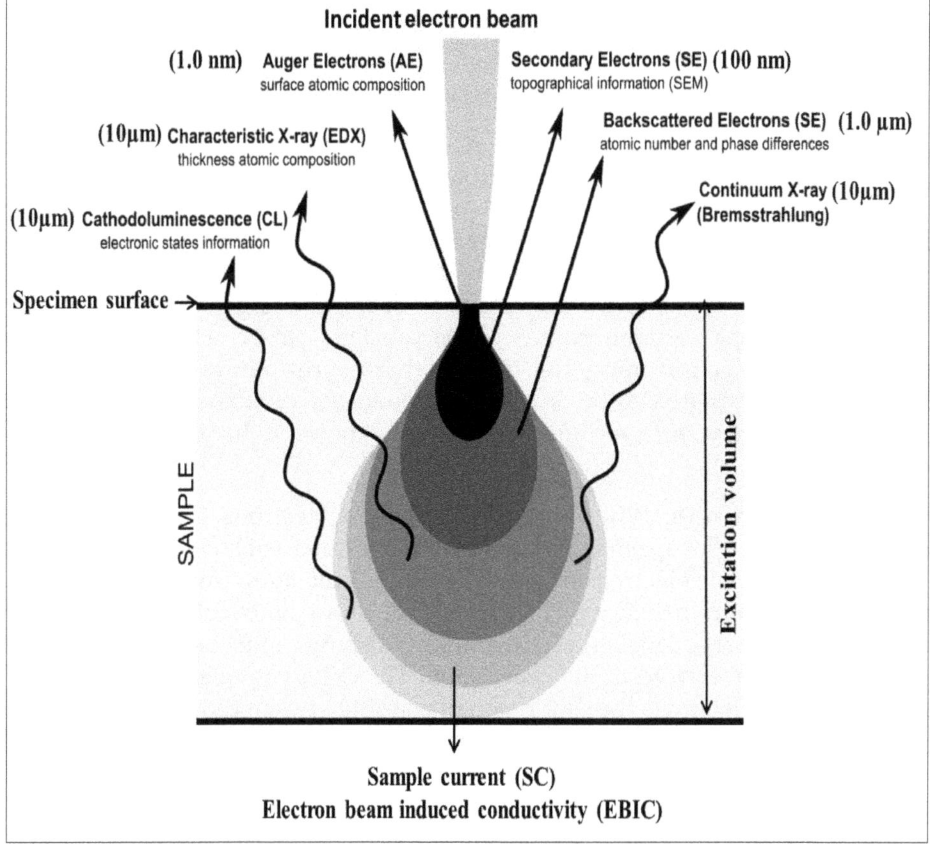

Backscattered electron: Those electrons, which are deflected, back in the direction of the beam. The special detector in scanning and transmission electron microscope traps these signals. These are used to discriminate areas of different atomic numbered elements. Higher atomic numbered elements gives off more backscattered electrons and appear brighter than lower numbered elements. It has the resolution to the level of 1000 nm. These electrons have high energy.

Secondary Electrons: These electrons are also collected with a special type of detector used in SEM. They are used primarily to reveal topographical feature of a specimen. It has the resolving power <10 nm. These electrons have low energy.

Auger Electrons: These are special types of low energy electrons that carry the information about the chemical nature (atomic composition) of the specimen. These are generated from the upper layer of specimen. It is a powerful tool in the material sciences for studying the distribution of the lighter numbered atomic elements on the surface of the specimen. It has limited application in biological sciences. It is specialized equipment known as scanning auger electron spectrometer.

Cathodoluminescent: This effect results when the energy of the impinging electrons in converted into visible light. Certain types of compounds are capable of cathode luminescence and detected by special types of detector. The resolution is the similar to the light microscope.

Bremsstrahlung: Two important types of x-ray may be generated when the beam electron encounters the atoms of the specimen, continuous or bremsstrahlung x-ray and characteristic x-ray are generated when incoming, beam passing close to the atomic nucleus is slowed by the coulomb field of the nucleus with the release of x- ray energy. The intensity of x-ray energy released depends on how close the electron comes to the nucleus closer. The closer passes decelerate the electron more and yield higher energy x-rays. These are used to measure specimen mass thickness when quantitative analysis performed on thin sections. These are continuous x-rays also known as background or white radiation.

Characteristic X-rays: When high energy beam electrons interact with the shell electrons of the specimen atoms so that an inner shell electron is ejected. The removal of this electron temporarily ionizes the atom until an outer shell electron drops into the vacancy to stabilize the atom. Since this electron comes from a higher energy level, a certain amount of energy must be given off before it will be accommodated in the inner shell. The energy is released as an x-ray, the energy which equals the difference in energy between the two shells. Since this x-ray is of a discrete energy level, rather than a continuous, this event may be plotted as discrete peaks. Different elements will fill the vacancies in shells in unique ways. This means that since each element will generate a unique series of peaks, the spectrum may be used to identify the elements; such discrete x-rays are termed characteristic x-rays. The equipment for detection x-rays are Energy Dispersive X-ray (EDX) detector and Wavelength Dispersive X-ray (WDX) Detector.

Sample preparation for SEM

Step	Chemical	Temperature	Time	Repetitions
Primary fixation	2.5% glutaraldehyde in distilled water	room or 0-4°C	2-4 hours or microwave	1
Wash	distilled water	room or 0-4°C	30 minutes	3-5
Secondary fixation	1-4% osmium tetroxide in distilled water	room or 0-4°C	2-4 hours	1
Wash	distilled water	room or 0-4°C	30 minutes	3-5
Dehydration	25% ethanol	room or 0-4°C	20 minutes	1
	50% ethanol		20 minutes	1
	70-75% ethanol		20 minutes	1
	90-95% ethanol		20 minutes	1
	100% ethanol		30 minutes	2

Critical point dry

Mount on specimen stub with silver paste or graphite

Sputtering coat the biological sample with gold/palladium alloy for making them conductive

Store stubs in desiccator and view the external surface with SEM

SEM Micrographs

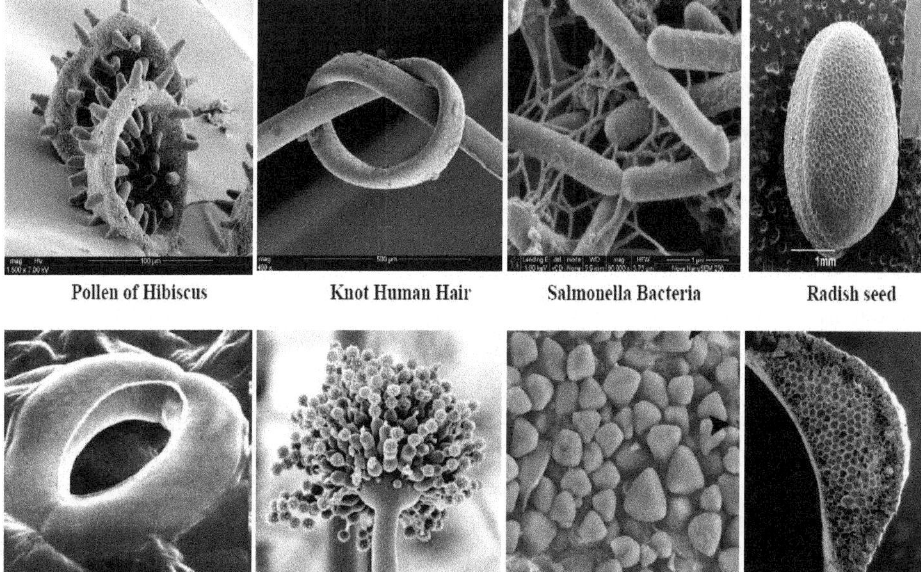

Pollen of Hibiscus | Knot Human Hair | Salmonella Bacteria | Radish seed

Guard cells | *Aspergillus niger* | Nuclear Polyhedrosis Virus | Cross section of leaf

Applications of Scanning Electron Microscopy

Topography: The surface features of an object or "how it looks", its texture; direct relation between these features and materials properties (hardness, reflectivity... etc.)

Morphology: The shape and size of the particles making up the object; direct relation between these structures and materials properties (ductility, strength, reactivity...etc.)

Composition: The elements and compounds that the object is composed of and the relative amounts of them; direct relationship between composition and materials properties (melting point, reactivity, hardness...etc.)

Crystallographic Information: How the atoms are arranged in the object; direct relation between these arrangements and materials properties (conductivity, electrical properties, strength.etc.)

Advantages of SEM

- It gives detailed 3D and topographical imaging and the versatile information garnered from different detectors.
- This instrument works very fast.
- Modern SEMs allow for the generation of data in digital form.
- Most SEM samples require minimal preparation actions.

Disadvantages of SEM

- SEMs are expensive and large.
- Special training is required to operate an SEM.
- The preparation of samples can result in artifacts.
- SEMs are limited to solid samples.
- SEMs carry a small risk of radiation exposure associated with the electrons that scatter from beneath the sample surface.

References

Goldstein, J.I., Yakowitz, H.. Newbury, D.E Lifshin, E.. Colby, J.W Colby J.W. and. J.R. Coleman. 1975. Pratical Scanning Electron Microscopy: Electron and Ion Microprobe Analysis.

Loretto, M.H. 1984. Electron Beam Analysis of Materials, in Chapman and Hall, London New York FEI. The Quanta 200 User's Operation Manual 2nd ed. (2004). I.M. Watt, The Principles and Practice of Electron Microscopy, (Cambridge Univ. Press. Cambridge, England, 1985.

Lyman, C.E., Newbury, D.E. Goldstein, J.I. Williams, D.B. Romig, A.D. Armstrong, J.T. Echlin, P.. Fiori, C.E Joy, D.C. Lifshin E.and Klaus-Ruediger Peters,

1990Scanning Electron Microscopy X-Ray Microanalysis and Analytical Electron Microscopy: A Laboratory Workbook, Press. New York, N.Y.

Postek, M.T.,. Howard, K.S Johnson A.H. McMichael K.L.1980. Scanning Electron Microscopy: A Student's Handbook, (Ladd Research Ind., Inc. Williston, VT.).

Self-assessment Questions

Fill in the blanks:

1. Electron microscope uses .... as a source for making images.
2. Electron microscope was invented by ....
3. Resolution of unaided human eye is ....
4. Primary fixative used in sample preparation of SEM is ....
5. Formula for Resolution is ....

Choose the correct answer

1. What is the resolving power of light microscope?
   - ii) 200 μm
   - iii) 0.02m
   - iv) 200nm
   - v) 0.2 mm
2. Which of the following is the first step in the processing of biological material for transmission electron microscopy?
   - i) Dehydration
   - ii) Sectioning
   - iii) Fixation
   - iv) Embedding
3. A vacuum is needed in the electron microscope to.......................................
   - i) Pull the electrons onto the specimen
   - ii) Eliminate molecules of nitrogen, oxygen or carbon dioxide
   - iii) Pull the specimen into the column
   - iv) Prevent secondary radiation affecting the microscope control panel
4. Which of the following statements about SEM is true?
   - i) The specimen is usually coated with gold
   - ii) Carbon nanotubes
   - iii) Quantum dots
   - iv) All the above
5. Ernst Ruska awarded Nobel prize during 1986 for their invention of______
   - i) SEM
   - ii) TEM
   - iii) STM
   - iv) AFM

True or False

1. Secondary electrons are formed by collision of incident beam and sample
2. In SEM copper grid is used as platform for sample analysis
3. Electron microscope was invented in the year 1931 by Max Knoll and Ernst Ruska.
4. In electron microscopy, the lenses used to magnify the image are made of glasses
5. 2.5% glutaraldehyde is used as primary fixative for SEM sample preparation

Short Notes

1. What is meant by backscattered electron
2. Light vs electron microscope differentiate
3. Why vacuum is needed in electron microscope?
4. Narrate the role of different components of SEM with illustration
5. Advantage and disadvantage of SEM?

Essay

1. Write in detail about essential components and working principle of scanning electron microscope with diagram

9

Transmission Electron Microscope: Principle, Components and Applications

Dr. M. Kannan

Transmission electron microscopy (TEM) is the original form of electron microscopy and analogues to the optical microscope. It can achieve a resolution of ~0.1 nm, thousand times better resolution, cannot be reached by the light microscope. The beam of electrons passes through the specimen and analyzes the internal structure of the specimen in the form of images. The electron has the poor penetrating capability and gets absorbed in the thick specimen. Therefore, the thickness of the specimen should not be more than few hundred Angstroms (one angtron = 10^{-10} m) However sometimes, slightly thickens samples are used in High Voltage Electron Microscope.

Components of TEM

Transmission electron microscope has three essential systems: (1) an electron gun, which produces the electron beam, and the condenser system, which focuses the beam onto the object (sample), (2) the image-producing system, consisting of the objective lens, movable specimen stage, objective, intermediate and projector lenses, which focus the electrons passing through the specimen to form a real, highly magnified image, and (3) the image-recording system, which converts the electron image into some form perceptible to the human eye. The image-recording system usually consists of a fluorescent screen for viewing and focusing the image and a digital CCD camera for permanent records. In addition, a vacuum system, consisting of pumps and their associated gauges and valves, and power supplies are required.

Illumination System (Electron gun and condenser lenses)

Electron Gun

The source of electrons, the cathode, is a heated a sharply pointed rod shaped lanthanum hexaboride (LaBb). The filament is surrounded by a control grid called as include Wehnelt cylinder, with a central aperture arranged on the axis of the column; the apex of the cathode is arranged to lie at or just above or below this aperture. The cathode and control grid are at a negative potential equal to the desired accelerating voltage and are insulated from the rest of the instrument. The final electrode of the electron gun is the anode, which takes the form of a disk with an axial hole. Electrons leave the cathode and accelerate toward the anode. The control and alignment of the electron gun are critical in ensuring satisfactory operation.

Condenser Lenses System

The intensity and angular aperture of the beam are controlled by the condenser lens system between the gun and the specimen. A single lens may be used to converge the beam onto the object, but, more commonly, a double condenser is employed. In this the first lens is strong and produces a reduced image of the source, which is then imaged by the second lens onto the object. The use of a small spot size minimizes disturbances in the specimen due to heating and irradiation.

The Image-producing System

Objective Lenses and Projector Lenses

The specimen grid is carried in a small holder in a movable specimen stage. The objective lens is usually of short focal length (1–5 mm) and produces a real intermediate image that is further magnified by the projector lens or lenses. A single projector lens may provide a range of magnification of 5:1, and by the use of interchangeable pole pieces in the projector a wider range of magnifications may be obtained. Modern instruments employ two projector lenses (one called the intermediate lens) to permit a greater range of magnification and to provide a greater overall magnification without a commensurate increase in the physical length of the column of the microscope.

For image stability and brightness, the microscope is often operated to give a final magnification of 1,000–250,000x on the screen. If a higher final magnification is required, it may be obtained by photographic or digital enlargement. The quality of the final image in the electron microscope depends largely upon the accuracy of the various mechanical and electrical adjustments with which the various lenses are aligned to one another and to the illuminating system. The lenses require power supplies of a high degree of stability; for the highest standard of resolution, electronic stabilization to better than one part in a million is necessary. The control of a modern electron microscope is carried out by a computer, and dedicated software is readily available.

Image Translation System (Fluorescent screen and Digital photographic unit)

TEM provides informations in the form of variations of electron intensity in the image. The electron image is monochromatic and must be made visible to the eye either by allowing the electrons to fall on a fluorescent screen fitted at the base of the microscope column or by capturing the image digitally for display on a computer monitor. Computerized images are stored in a format such as TIFF or JPEG.

How Transmission Electron Microscopy (TEM) Works

TEM involves a high voltage electron beam emitted from a tungsten filament (cathode) by electrical heating; the shaft of electrons beam drawn toward an anode (magnetic lenses) and pass through an aperture. The beam traverses the aperture and next moves through an electromagnetic condenser, objective, intermediate and projector lens. The focused electron beam transmitted through a very thin specimen (50nm size, semitransparent for electrons and carries information about the structure of the specimen) loaded on a grid inserted in the path and manipulated by goniometer. The part of the beam absorbed scattered and transmitted through objective aperture and projected by projector lens after corrected by intermediate lenses on the fluorescence screen. The image is observed with the help of optical binocular attached to its viewing window. The spatial variation in the "image" is then magnified by a series of magnetic lenses until it is recorded by hitting a fluorescent screen or light sensitive sensor such as a CCD (charge-coupled device) camera fitted either in the side or bottom of the photographic plate. TEM electron scattering rather than differences in absorbance produces contrast in the image. Scattering results from an interaction between specimen atoms and electrons of the illuminating beam. The negatively charged electron clouds around atomic nuclei scatter electrons by repelling them. These effects increase as electrons pass closer to specimen atoms. Nuclei of high atomic number, as in atom of heavy metals such as lead and uranium, cause a widest scattering. Transmission electron microscopes produce two-dimensional, black and white images. The TEM can easily resolve structure such as ribosome, microtubules, microfilaments and large molecules such as proteins. Even images of individual heavy metal atom have been produced under the special operating conditions.

Transmission Electron Microscopy (TEM)

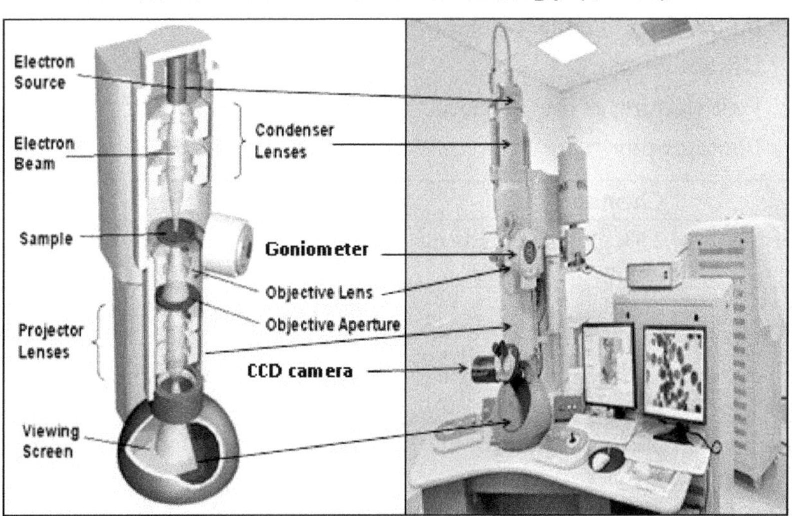

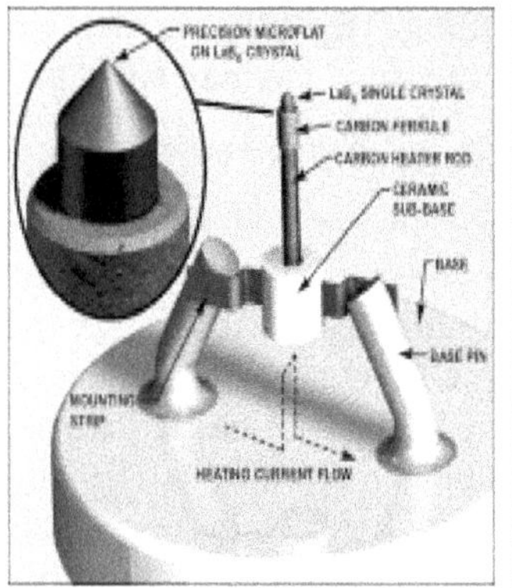

Electron gun source LB 6

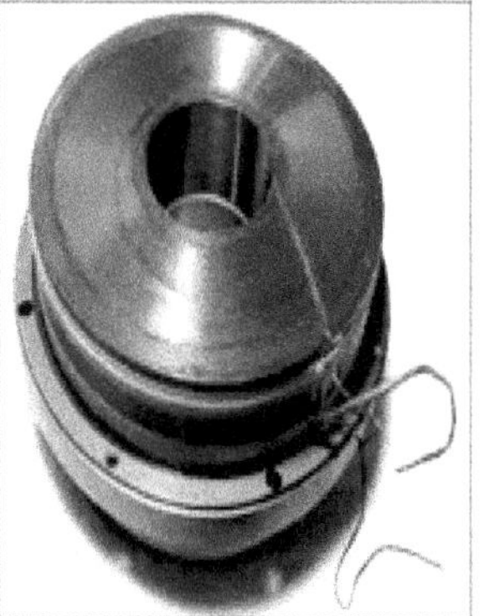

Electromagnetic lens

TEM specimen holder

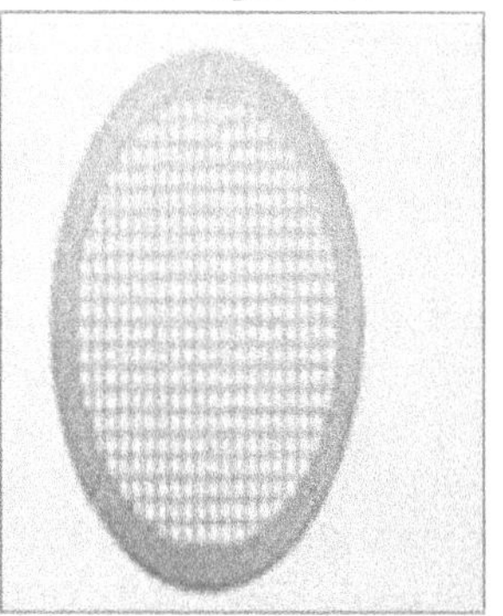

TEM Copper grid mesh

Biological Sample Preparation Techniques for TEM

1. Tissue isolation
2. Fixation with glutaraldehyde, OsO_4 and occasionally $KMnO_4$
3. Embedding in a plastic resin
4. Ultramicrotomy
5. Post-staining of thin sections
6. Photography

tep	Chemical	Temperature	Time	Repetitions
Primary fixation	2.5% glutaraldehyde in buffer	room or 0-4°C	2-4 hours or microwave	1
Wash	buffer	room or 0-4°C	30 minutes	3-5
Secondary fixation	1-4% osmium tetroxide in buffer	room or 0-4°C	2-4 hours	1
Wash	buffer or distilled water	room or 0-4°C	30 minutes	3-5

en bloc staining (optional)	0.5% uranyl acetate	0-4°C	overnight	1
Wash after *en bloc* staining	distilled water	room or 0-4°C	10-15 minutes	2
Dehydration	25% ethanol 50% ethanol 70-75% ethanol 90-95% ethanol 100% ethanol Transition solvent if embedding resin is not miscible with ethanol	room or 0-4°C	20 minutes 20 minutes 20 minutes 20 minutes 30 minutes	1 1 1 1 2
Infiltration	1 part resin/2 parts solvent 1 part resin/1 part solvent (optional) 2 parts resin/1 part solvent 100% resin	room room room room	1 hour-overnight 1 hour-overnight 1 hour-overnight 1 hour	1 1 1 1
Embedding	Place in 100% resin in suitable container	1	1	11
Degassing (optional)	Place in vacuum desiccator or vacuum oven	room-60° C	3-30 minutes	
Polymerization	Place in vacuum desiccator or vacuum oven	60-70° C	> 8 hours	
Ultramicrotomy	• Trimming the capsule • Making glass knives • Sectioning - Thick sections (500nm size) - light microscopy - Thin sections (50nm size) - TEM • Staining sections - Thick sections – Toluidine blue staining light microscopy - Thin sections (50nm size) – Negative staining using 1-2% Phosphotungstic acid (PTA) or uranyl acetate or Bacteria, virus, bacteriophages and cell fragment samples • Photography - Capturing the image from thin section			

Ultramicrotomy of processed biological samples

Ultramicrotome

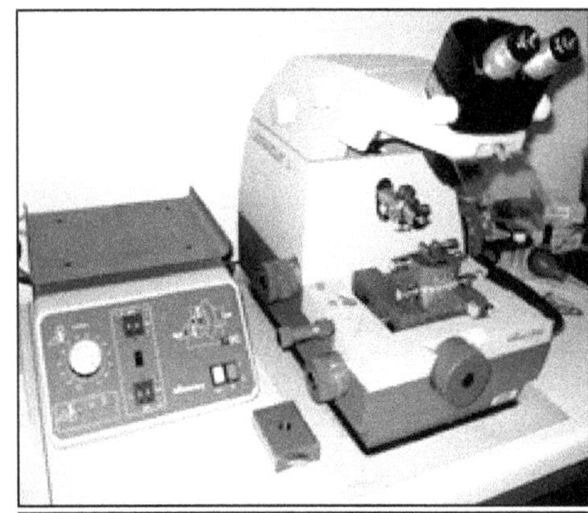

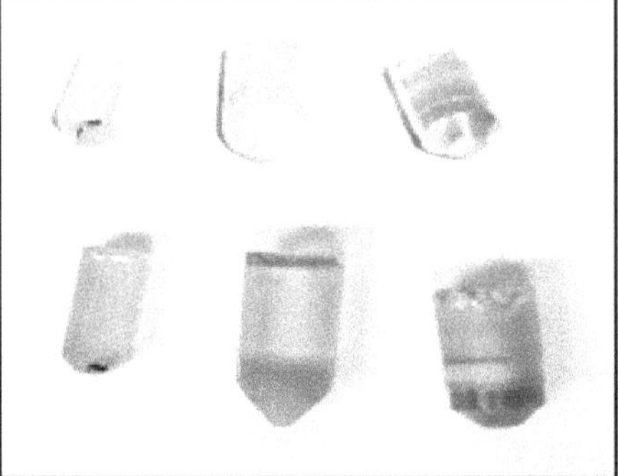

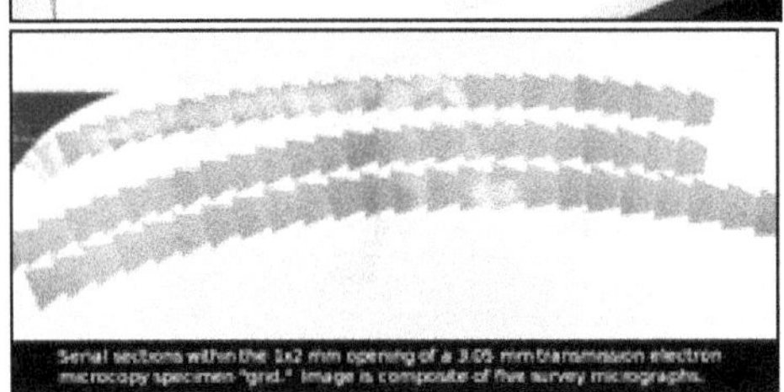

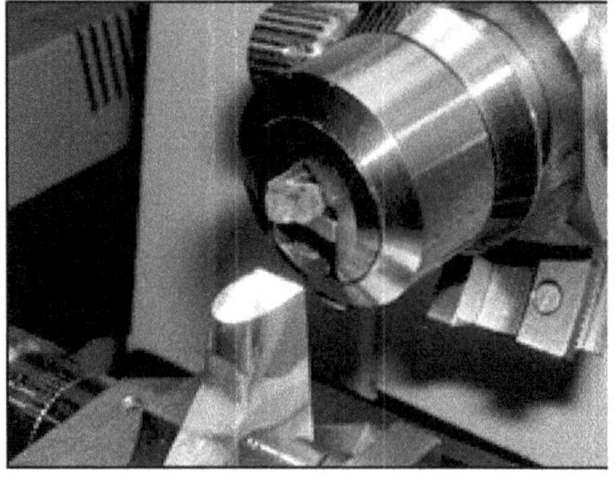

TEM of Plant cell ultra structure

Cytoplasm

Vacuole

Starch granules

Chloroplast

mitochondrion

Cell wall

Chromosomes

Nuclear membrane

Endoplasmic reticulum

Plasma membrane

TEM micrographs of plant cell organelles

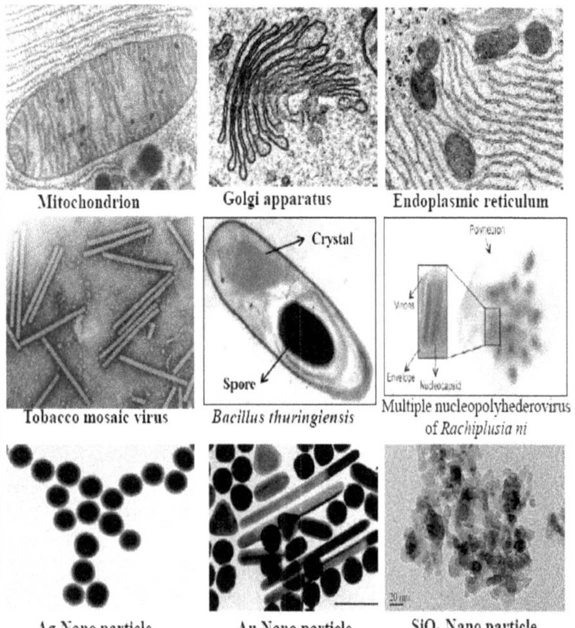

Ag Nano particle

Au Nano particle

SiO_2 Nano particle

Difference Between TEM and SEM

Sl. No.	Feature	TEM	SEM
1.	Electron Beam	Broad, static beams	Beam focused to fine point; sample is scanned line by line
2.	Voltages Needed	Accelerating voltage much lower; not necessary to penetrate the specimen	SEM voltage ranges from 60-300,000 volts
3.	Interaction of the beam electrons	Specimen must be very thin	Wide range of specimens allowed; simplifies sample preparation
4.	Imaging	Electrons must pass through and be transmitted by the specimen	Information needed is collected near the surface of the specimen
5.	Image Rendering	Transmitted electrons are collectively focused by the objective lens and magnified to create a real image	Beam is scanned along the surface of the sample to build up the image

Application of TEM

- Transmission Electron Microscope is ideal for a number of different fields such as life sciences, nanotechnology, medical, biological and material research, forensic analysis, gemology and metallurgy as well as industry and education.
- TEMs provide topographical, morphological, compositional and crystalline information.
- The images allow researchers to view samples on a molecular level, making it possible to analyze structure and texture.
- This information is useful in the study of crystals and metals, but also has industrial applications.
- TEMs can be used in semiconductor analysis and production and the manufacturing of computer and silicon chips.
- Technology companies use TEMs to identify flaws, fractures and damages to micro-sized objects; this data can help fix problems and/or help to make a more durable, efficient product.
- Colleges and universities can utilize TEMs for research and studies.
- Although electron microscopes require specialized training, students can assist professors and learn TEM techniques.
- Students will have the opportunity to observe a nano-sized world in incredible depth and detail.

Advantages

- TEMs offer the most powerful magnification, potentially over one million times or more
- TEMs have a wide-range of applications and can be utilized in a variety of different scientific, educational and industrial fields
- TEMs provide information on element and compound structure
- Images are high-quality and detailed
- TEMs are able to yield information of surface features, shape, size and structure
- They are easy to operate with proper training

Disadvantages

- Some cons of electron microscopes include:
- TEMs are large and very expensive
- Laborious sample preparation
- Potential artifacts from sample preparation
- Operation and analysis requires special training
- Samples are limited to those that are electron transparent, able to tolerate the vacuum chamber and small enough to fit in the chamber
- TEMs require special housing and maintenance
- Images are black and white
- Electron microscopes are sensitive to vibration and electromagnetic fields and must be housed in an area that isolates them from possible exposure.
- A TEM requires constant upkeep including maintaining voltage, currents to the electromagnetic coils and cooling water.

References

Fultz, B. and. Howe, J.M. 2001. Transmission Electron Microscopy and Diffractometry of Materials, , Springer-Verlag Berlin Heidelberg New York.

Goldstein, J.I., Yakowitz, H.. Newbury, D.E Lifshin, E.. Colby, J.W Colby J.W. and. J.R. Coleman. 1975. Pratical Scanning Electron Microscopy: Electron and Ion Microprobe Analysis.

Thomas, G. J. Michael and Goringe. 1979. Transmission Electron Microscopy of Materials, A Wiley-Interscience Publication, USA.

Self-assessment Questions

Fill in the blank:

1. In tem ______________ is used as platform to keep the sample for imaging
2. TEM uses ______________ as a source for making images.
3. TEM imaging sample sectioning done by______________.
4. Thickness of the sample for TEM imaging is ______________.
5. ______________ and ______________ are used for negative staining of sample for TEM

Choose the correct answer

1. What is the resolving power of the Electron microscope?
   1. 100 nm
   2. 1.0 μm
   3. 0.05 nm
   4. 50 nm
2. 2. Sample is supported with ______________ for transmission electron microscope?
   1. Copper
   2. Gold plates
   3. Glass slide
   4. Thin film
3. Which of the following is not an advantage of TEM? ----------------.
   1. High resolution
   2. Samples for TEM can be chemically fixed
   3. High magnification
   4. Thin sections of tissue are not necessary
4. 4. Plant viruses can be seen through ______________ microscope
   1. SEM
   2. STM
   3. TEM
   4. AFM
5. We can see the internal content of the sample in the
   1. TEM
   2. Light microscope
   3. SEM
   4. All the above

True or False

1. Electrons flow away from the filament because of the large voltage difference between the filament and the anode plate
2. In electron microscopy, the lenses used to magnify the image are made of electromagnets

3. The difference between TEM and SEM is that in TEM, secondary low energy electrons are used to produce an image.
4. Negative staining is required for processing of virus sample in TEM
5. 1000 nm thickness sectioning of sample is sufficient for TEM imaging

Short notes

1. Applications of TEM
2. Working principle of TEM.
3. Differentiate TEM vs SEM
4. Write the biological sample preparation protocol for TEM imaging?
5. Explain the role of different components of TEM?

Essay

1. Write in detail about essential components and working principle and application of TEM

Dimensions
100 µm
Plant,
Animal Cell
10 µm
Bacteria
1 µm
100 nm
Virus
Protein
10 nm
DNA "turn"
Simple
Molecules
1 nm
DNA "base"
Atoms
0.1 nm

(P. 2)

The Role of Surface Area
Each side = 1 meter
Each side = ¼ meter
Each side = 1 nanometer
Gold
1 m
¼ m
Mass ≈ 43,000 lb
SA = 6 m²
Mass ≈ 43,000 lb
SA = 24 m²
Mass ≈ 43,000 lb
SA ≈ 6 billion m²
≈ 2500 sq miles
≈ 8 ft x 8 ft room
State of Delaware:
< 2000 sq miles
Policy question: Should regulation/risk assessment be based on mass or volume or on surface area/# of particles?
RICE

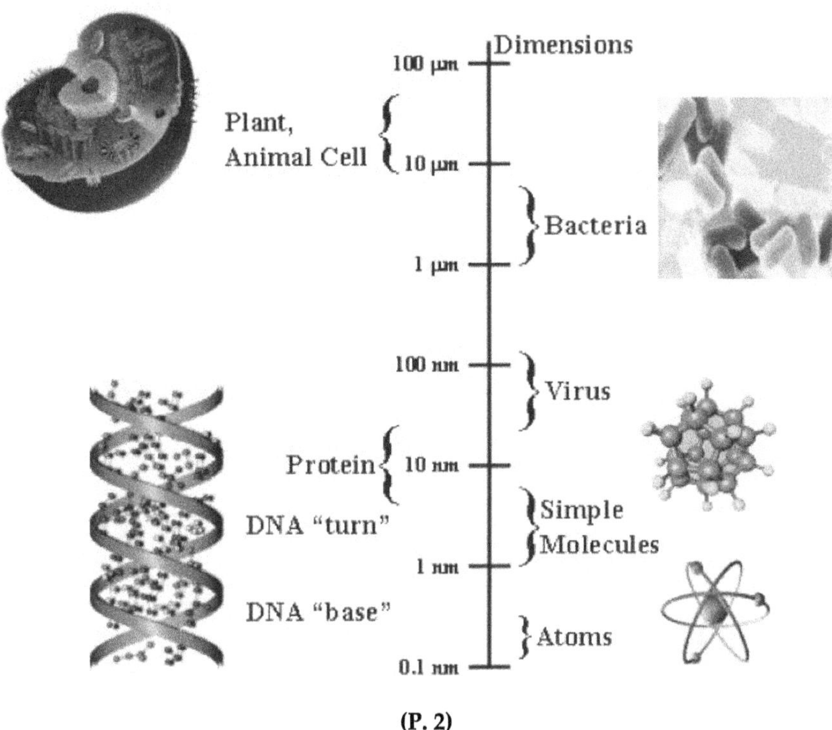

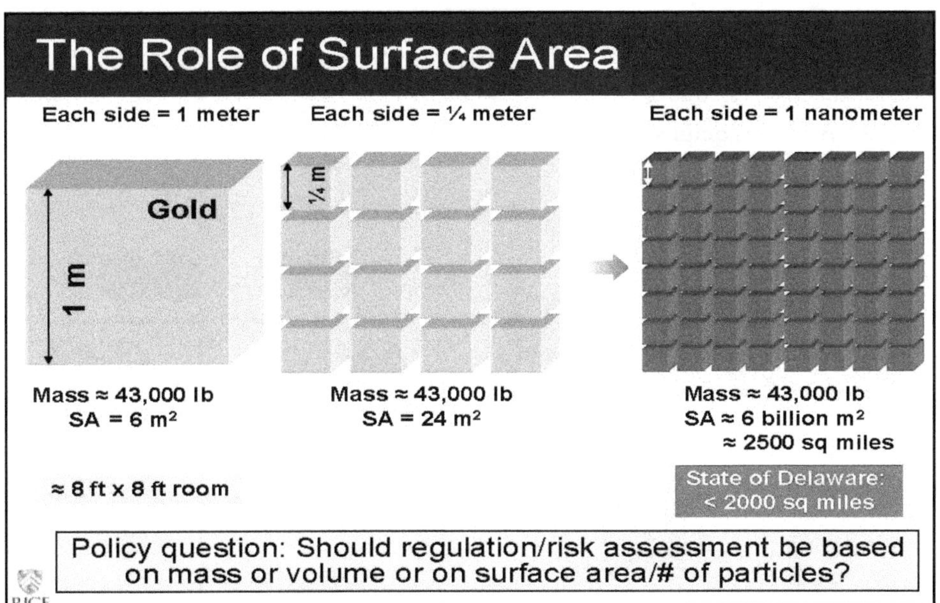

(P. 6)

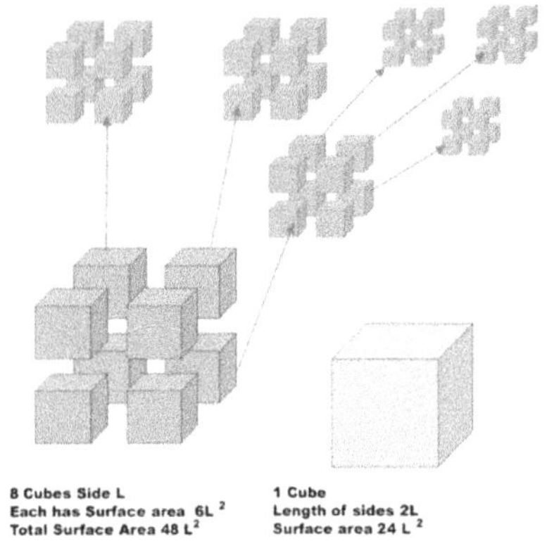

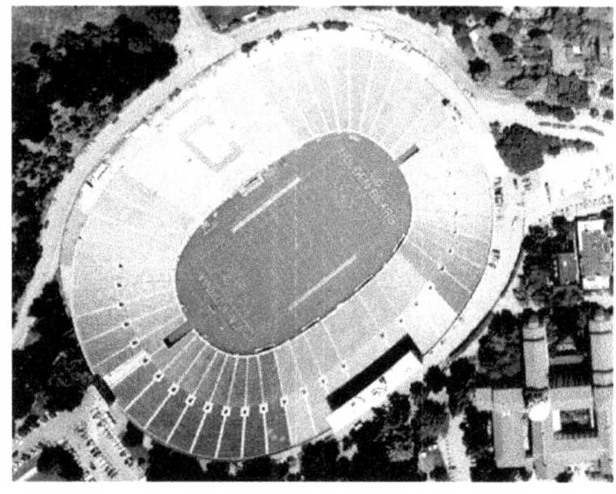

(P. 6)

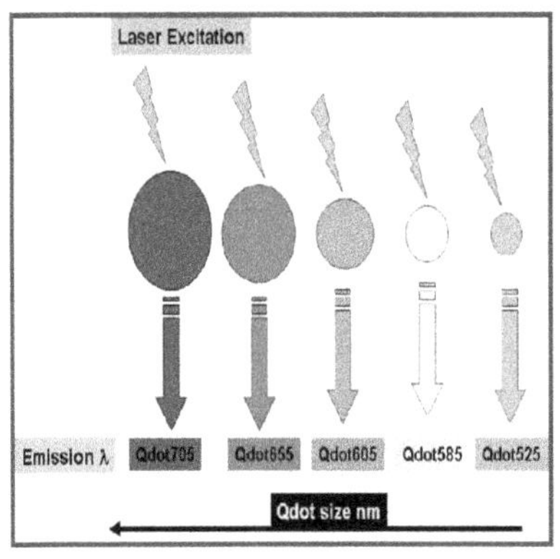

Fig. 3 [www.icms.qmul.ac] (P. 17)

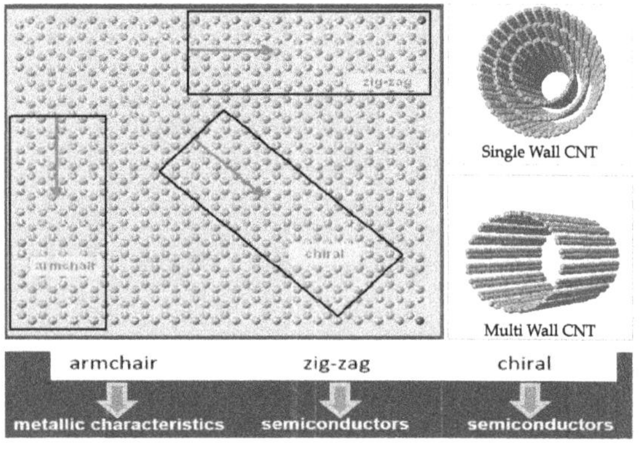

Fig. 6 [academic.pgcc.edu] (P. 19)

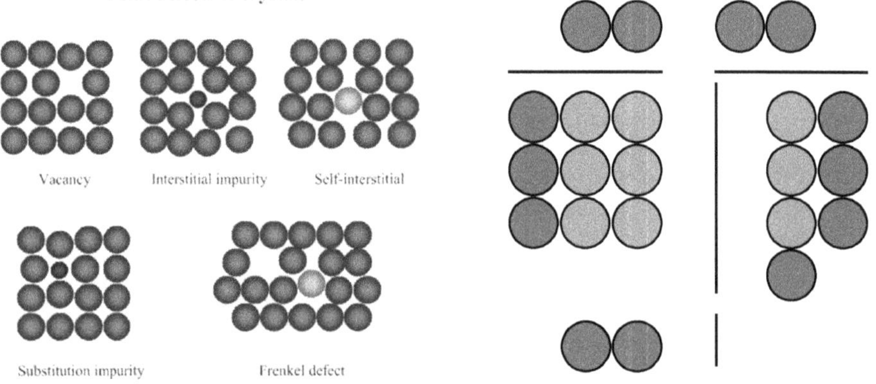

Fig. 3.1 (P. 21)

Fig. 5 (P. 24)

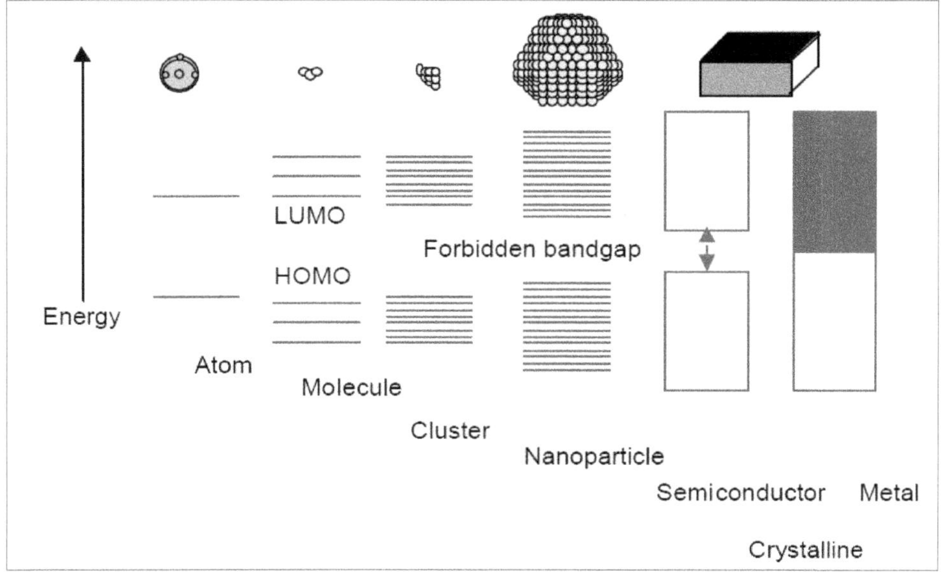

Fig. 10 (P. 28)

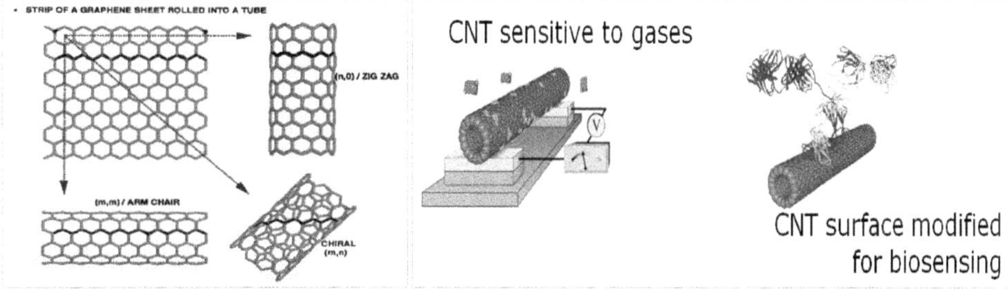

Fig 11 a & b (P. 29)

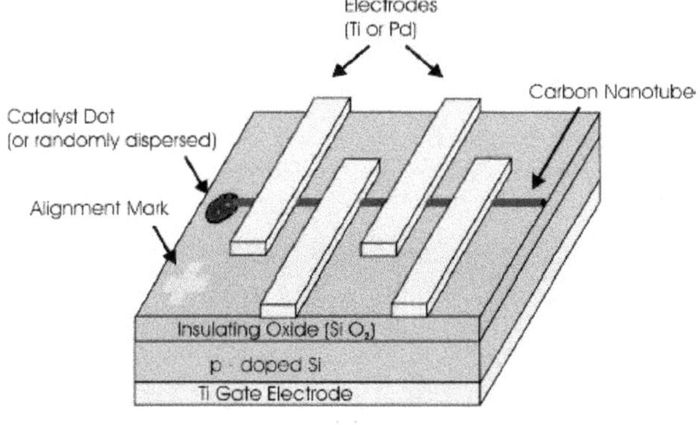

Fig. 12 (P. 30)

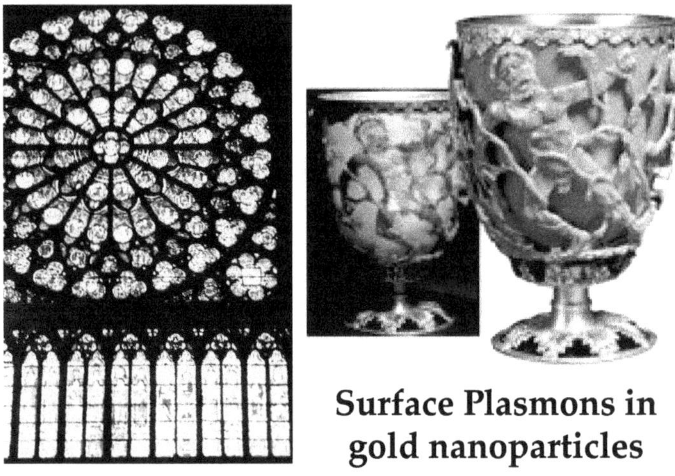

Fig. 13 a & b (P. 30)

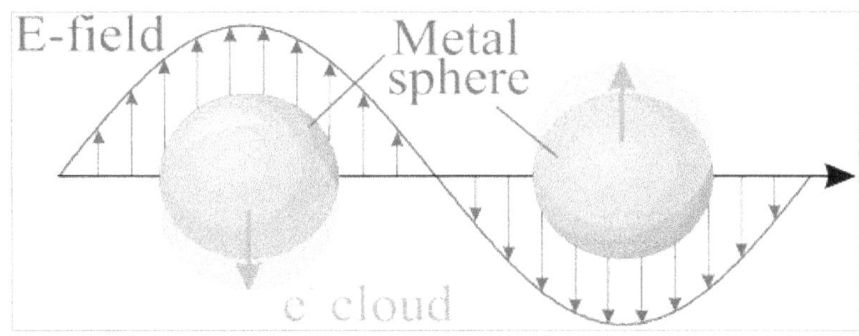

Fig. 14 (P. 31)

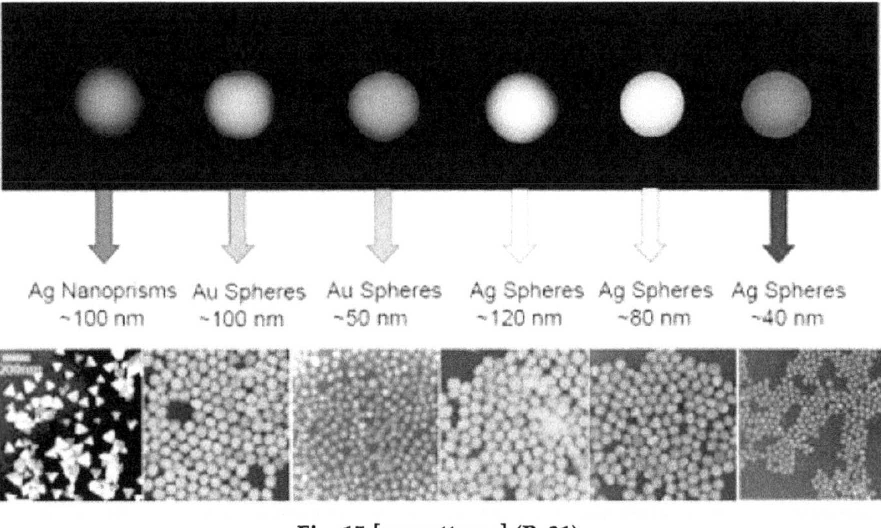

Fig. 15 [www.ttu.ee] (P. 31)

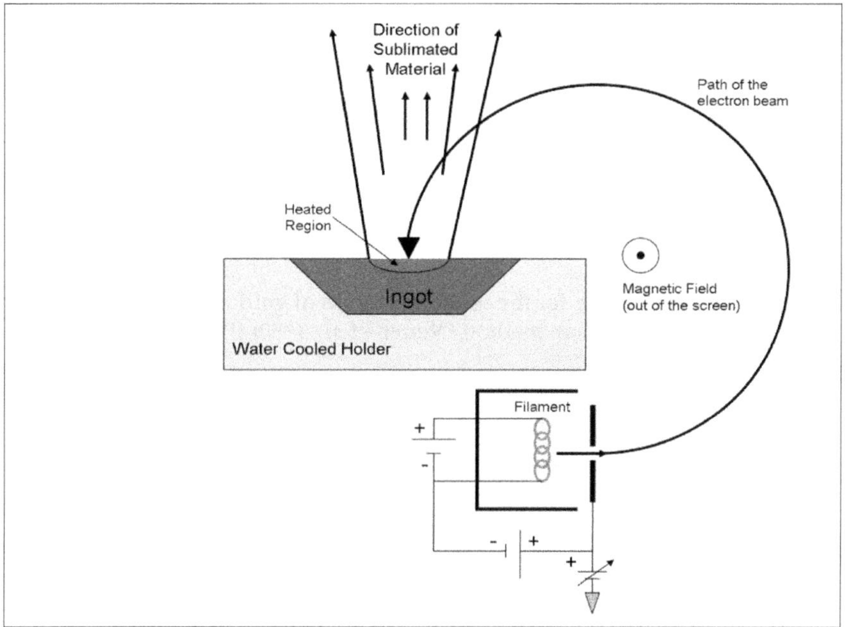

Fig. 2: Electron beam evaporation unit where ingot (evaporant) is positioned over hearth with water cooling mechanism and filament is used to generate electrons directed through magnetic field to the ingot location **(P. 36)**

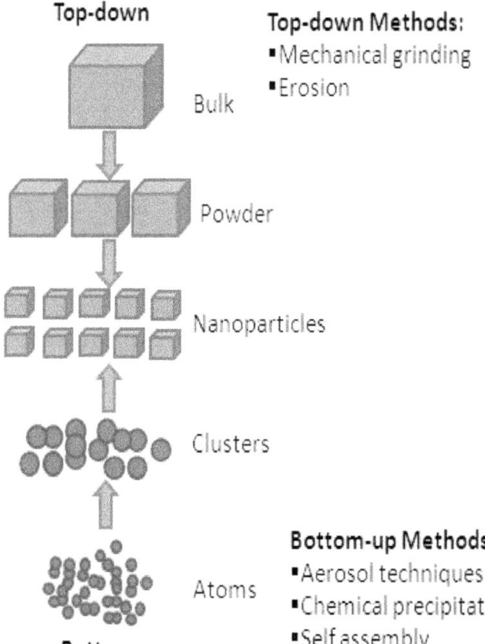

Fig. 1: Schematic diagram of top down and bottom up approaches **(P. 45)**

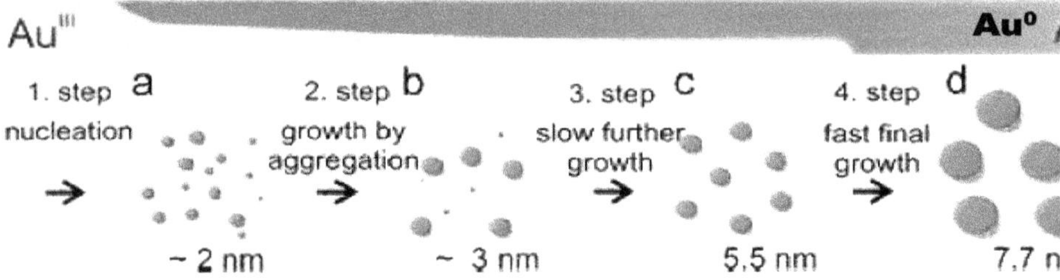

Fig. 3: Schematic diagram for the reduced process of gold nanoparticle formation reduction method (Nguen *et al.*, 1950) (P. 47)

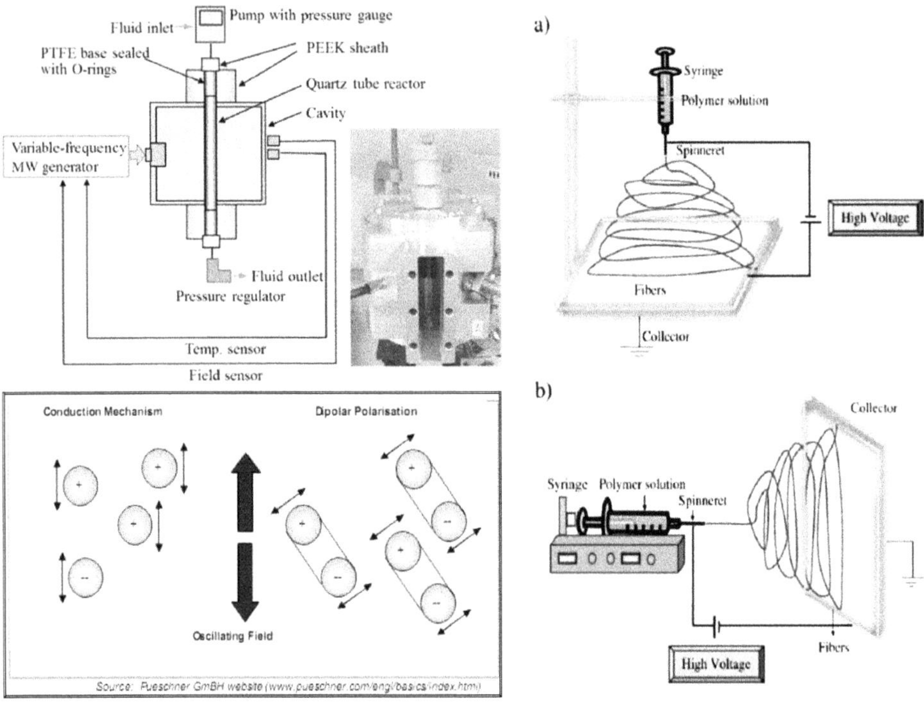

Fig. 6: Microwave apparatus set up and dipolar polarization and ionic conduction (P. 51)

Fig. 7a &b. Electrospinning set up (P. 53)

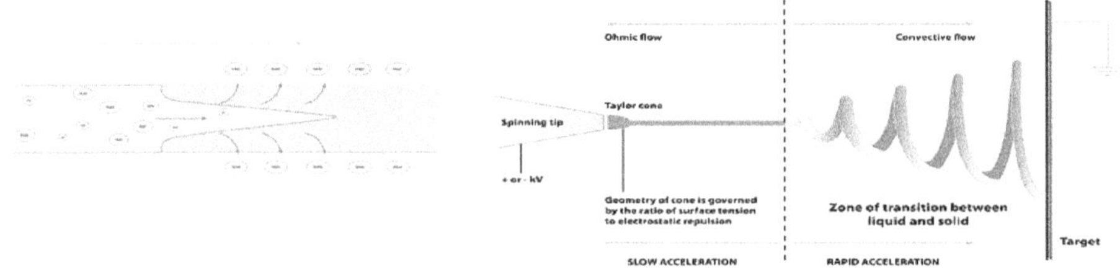

Fig. 8: Tayler cone and fibre formation by electrospinning (P. 53)

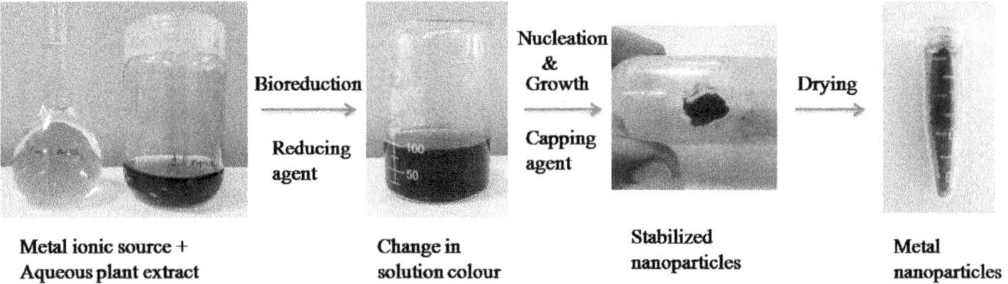

Fig. 2: Steps involved in biological synthesis of silver nanoparticles using dried leaf extract of *Andrographis paniculata* (Photo: Haripriya Shanmugam). (P. 62)

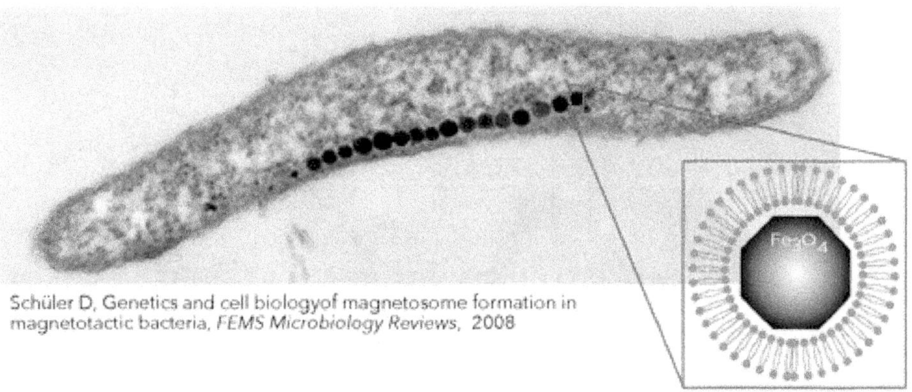

Fig. 3: Magnetosomes synthesized by magnetotactic bacteria (P. 64)

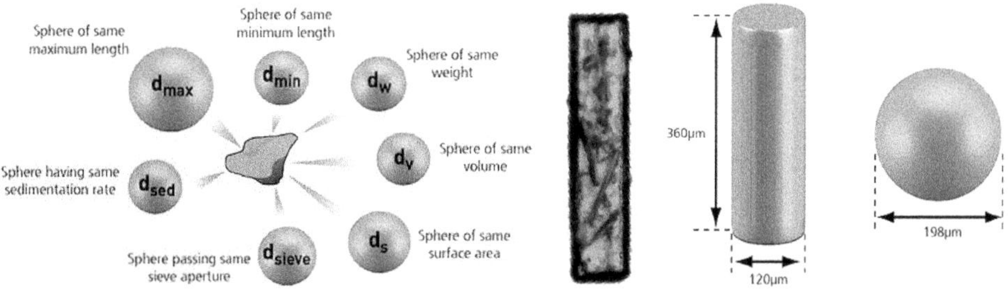

Fig. 1: Concept of equivalent sphere (P. 70)

Fig. 2: Volume equivalent rod and sphere of a needle shaped particle (P. 70)

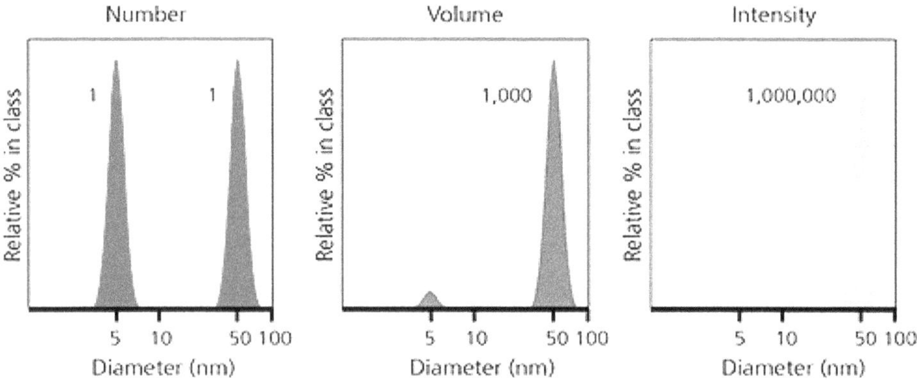

Fig. 3: Example of number, volume and intensity weighted particle size distributions for the same sample (P. 72)

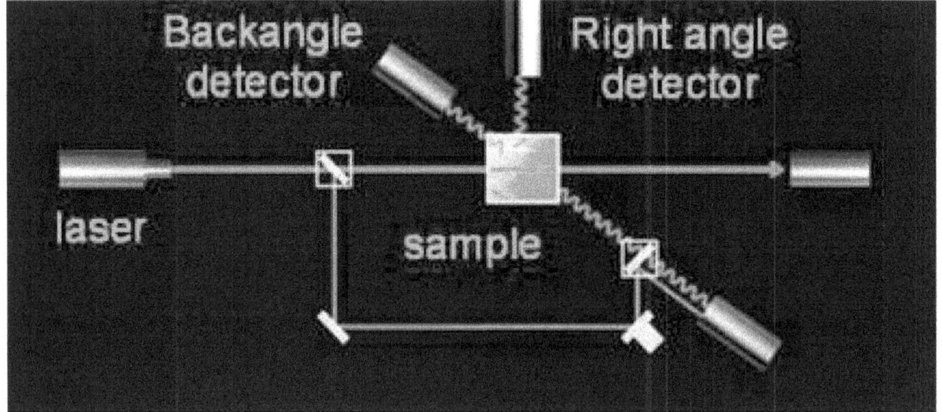

Fig. 7: Optical setup for dynamic light scattering (DLS) nanoparticle size analyzer (P. 77)

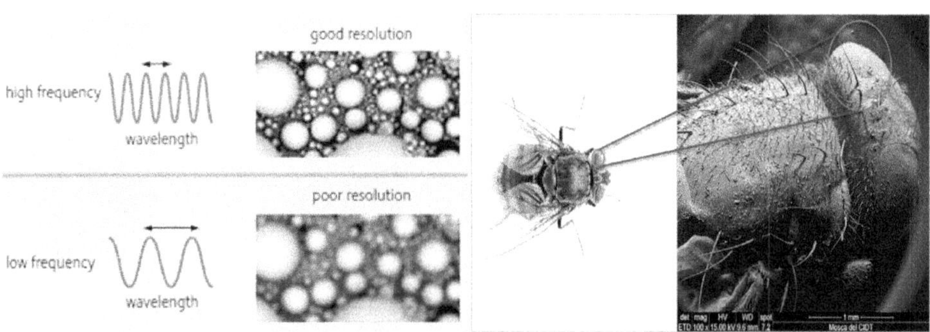

Resolution **Magnification**

(P. 82)

light microscope
objective lens
light beam
specimen
light source

TEM
electron source
first condenser lens
second condenser lens
condenser aperture
objective condenser lens
objective aperture
minicondenser lens
specimen (thin)
selected area aperture
objective imaging lens
diffraction lens
intermediate lens
first projector lens
second projector lens
projection chamber
fluorescent screen

SEM
electron source
anode
gun align coils
lens 1
lens 2
electron beam
scan & stig coils
lens 3
collector system
secondary electrons
electron beam impact area
specimen (thick)
vacuum
turbo/diff pump
roughing line

(P. 83)

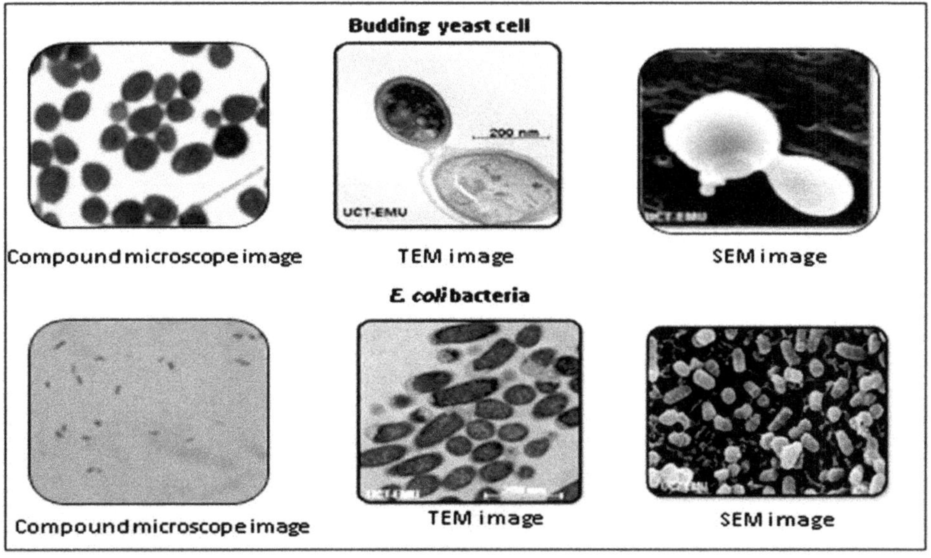

(P. 83)

Scanning Electron Microscope (SEM)
electron gun
electron beam
accelerating anode
focusing magnet
to screen control
scanning magnet
backscattered electron detector
X-ray detector
secondary electron detecto
sample
sample stage
EDAX

Thermionic Emission Gun
LaB_6 (Lanthanum hexaboride)
Field Emission Gun
Electromagnetic Lenses

(P. 85)

Detectors
X-rays: Energy dispersive spectrometer (EDS)
Secondary electron detector: (Everhart-Thornley)
Backscattered electron detector:(Solid-State Detector)

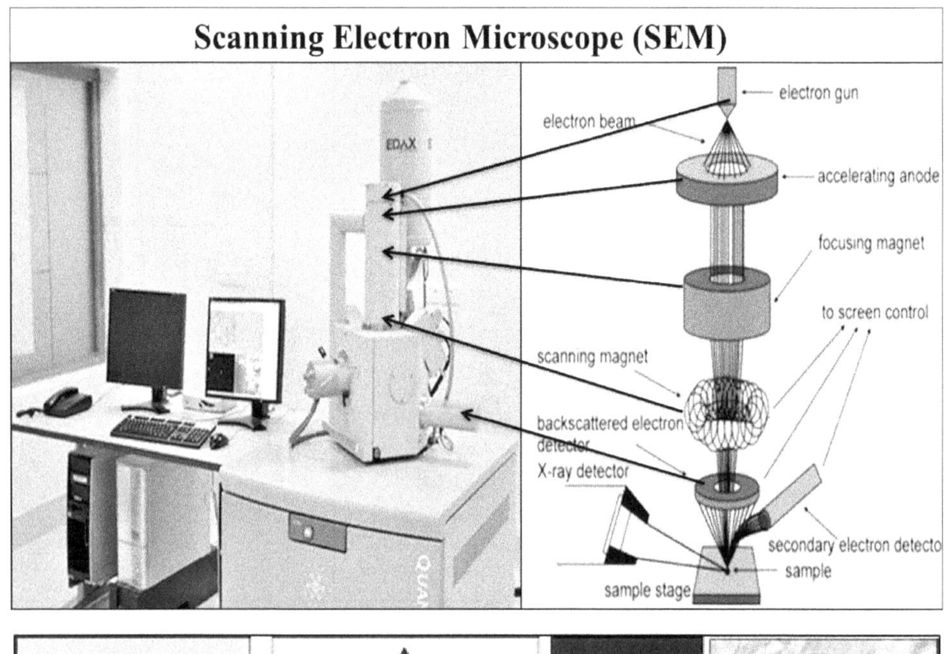

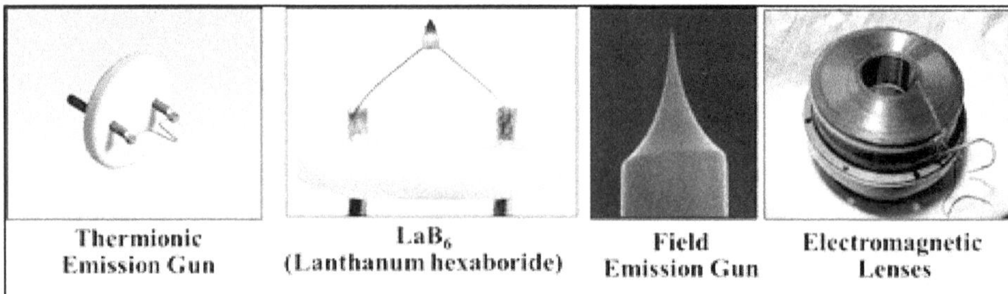

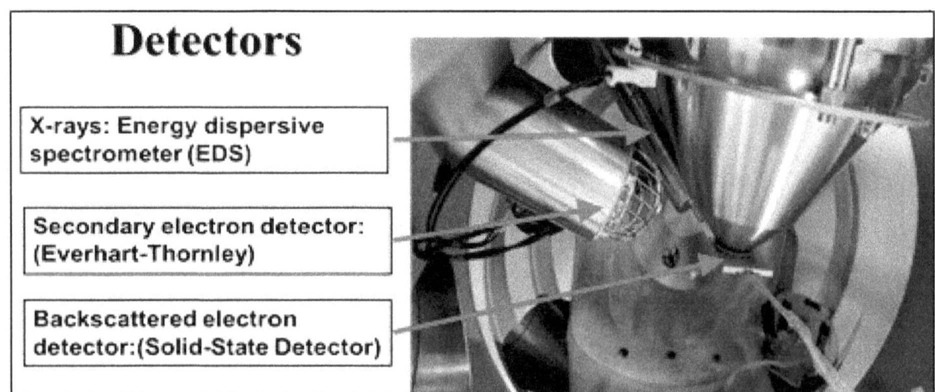

(P. 86)

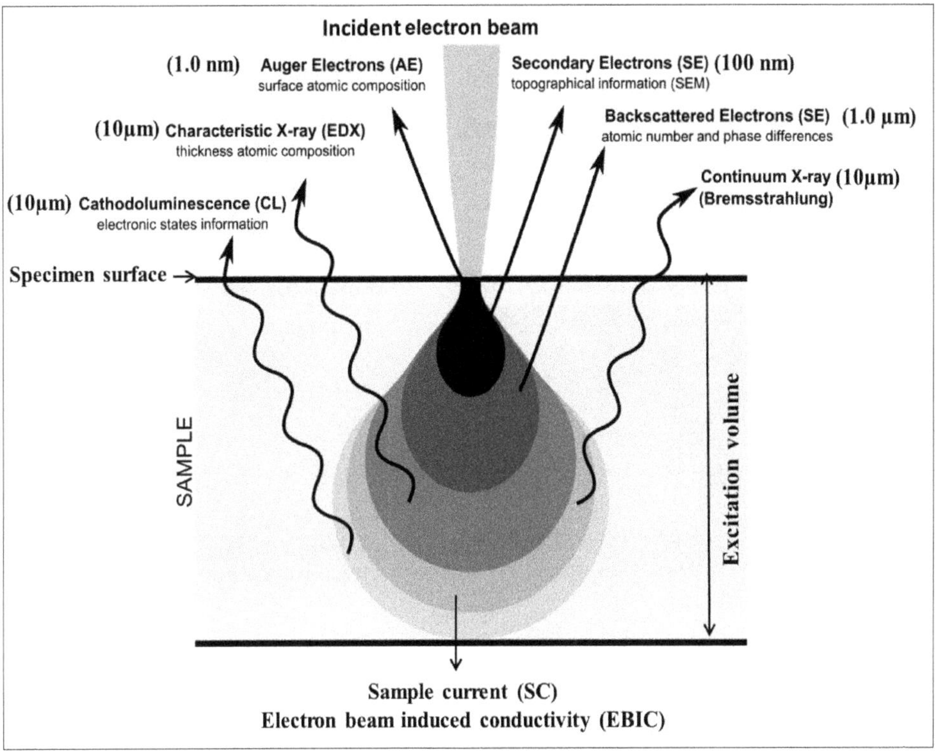

Incident electron beam
(1.0 nm) Auger Electrons (AE)
surface atomic composition
Secondary Electrons (SE) (100 nm)
topographical information (SEM)
(10μm) Characteristic X-ray (EDX)
thickness atomic composition
Backscattered Electrons (SE) (1.0 μm)
atomic number and phase differences
Continuum X-ray (10μm)
(Bremsstrahlung)
(10μm) Cathodoluminescence (CL)
electronic states information
Specimen surface
SAMPLE
Excitation volume
Sample current (SC)
Electron beam induced conductivity (EBIC)

(P. 87)

Transmission Electron Microscopy (TEM)

Electron Source
Electron Beam
Condenser Lenses
Sample
Goniometer
Objective Lens
Objective Aperture
Projector Lenses
CCD camera
Viewing Screen

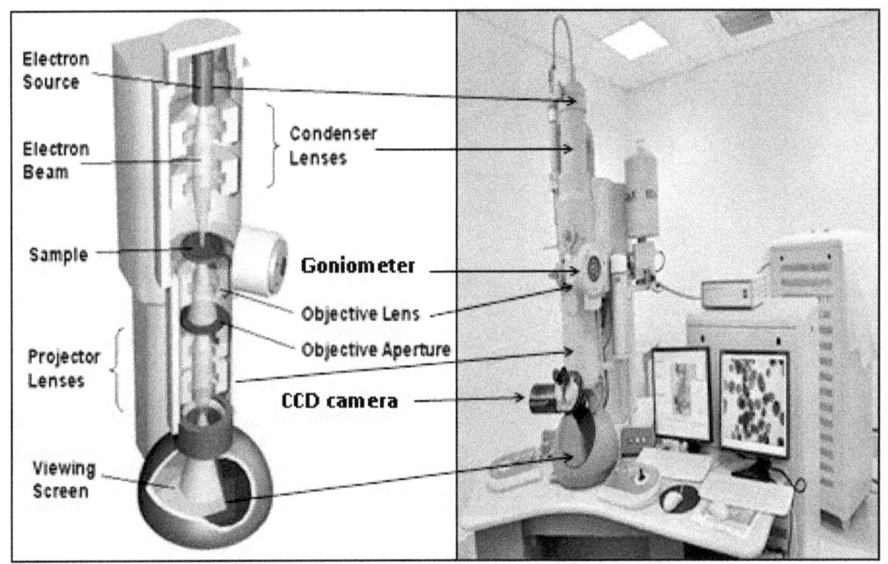

(P. 95)

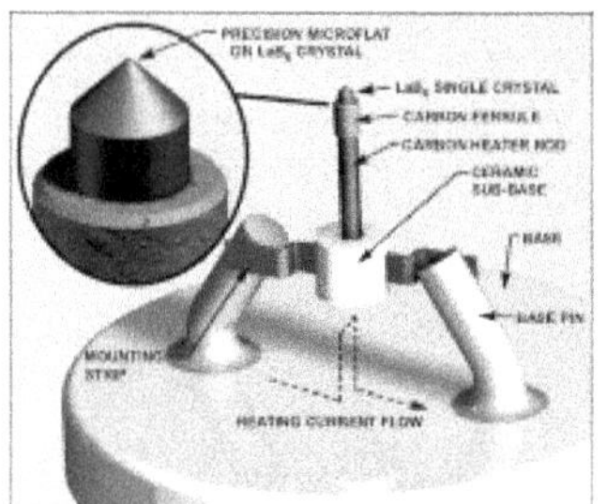

Electron gun source LB 6

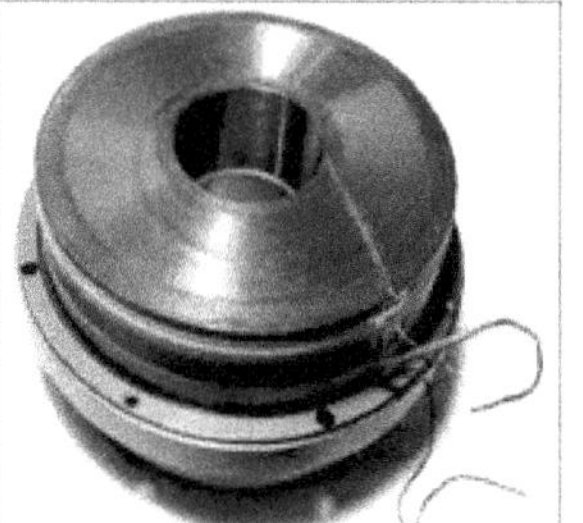

Electromagnetic lens

10mm
electron-beam
B-field
specimen-slot
electric connections
pulsed-field TEM specimen holder

TEM specimen holder

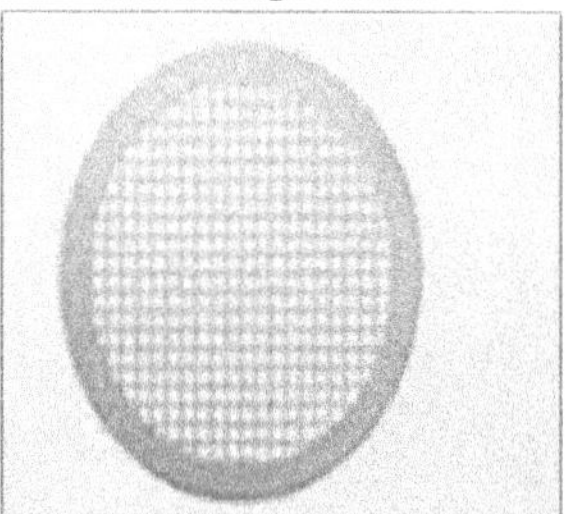

TEM Copper grid mesh

(P. 96)

Ultramicrotome

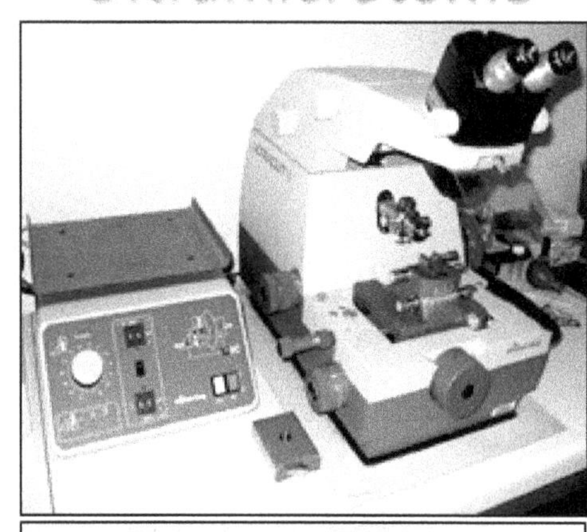

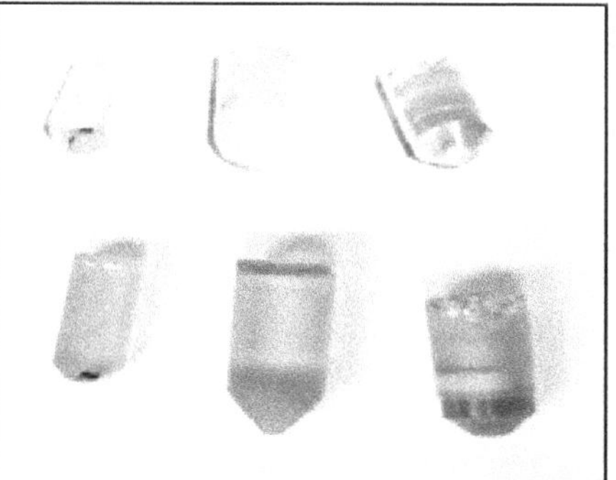

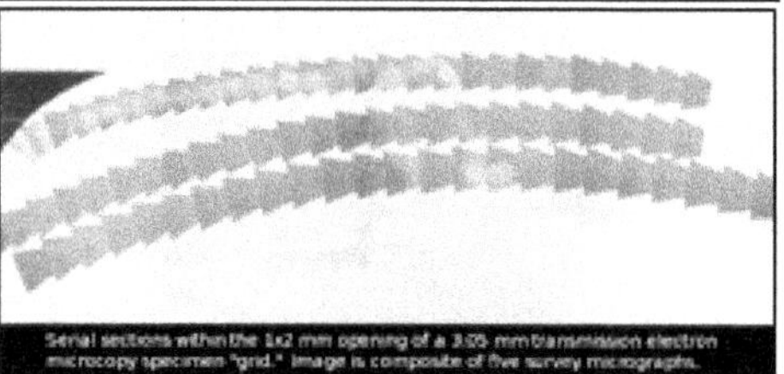

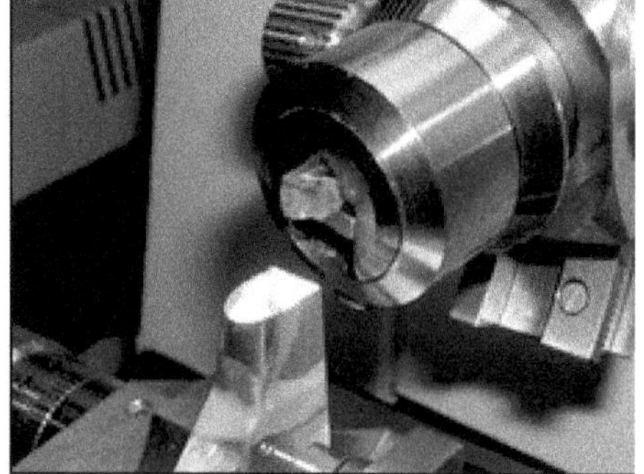

(P. 98)

10

UV: Vis Spectroscopy

Dr Pon. Sathya Moorthy

Spectroscopy

Spectroscopy is the study of the interaction between matter and electromagnetic radiation (Fig: 1). Any interaction with radiative energy is a function of its **wavelength or frequency**. Absorption occurs when energy from the radiative source is **absorbed by the material.** Emission indicates that radiative **energy released** by the material. The patterns of absorption and/or emission are called **spectra**. Spectra serve as a finger print for the nature of the sample and its chemical environment. Few examples for absorption spectroscopic methods are colorimetry, UV-Vis spectroscopy, Infrared spectroscopy, Nuclear magnetic resonance (NMR), Atomic absorption spectroscopy (AAS). Whereas, Fluorimetry, Flame photometry, *etc.*, are some example for emission spectroscopy.

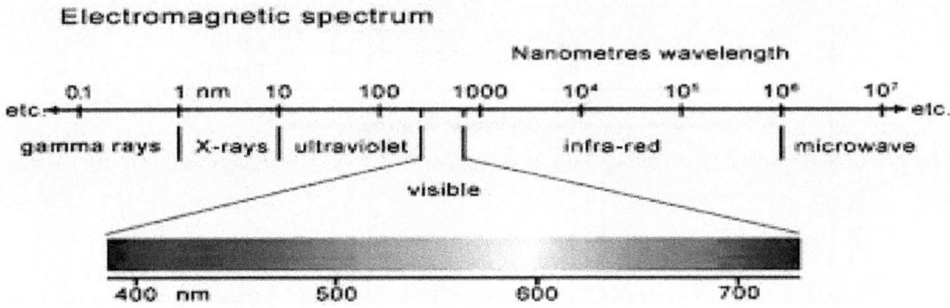

Fig. 1: Electromagnetic spectra in terms of wavelength (λ)

UV-Vis Spectroscopy

Ultraviolet (UV) and visible radiation comprise only a small part of the electromagnetic spectrum, ranges from **190 - 780 nm**. When UV-Vis radiation falls on the sample, a particular frequency of radiation gets readily absorbed due to their nature and its chemical environment. Many organic molecules which absorb only particular frequency of UV-Vis radiation due to the presence of certain **functional group**. Such function groups are termed as **Chromophores** (Fig.2).

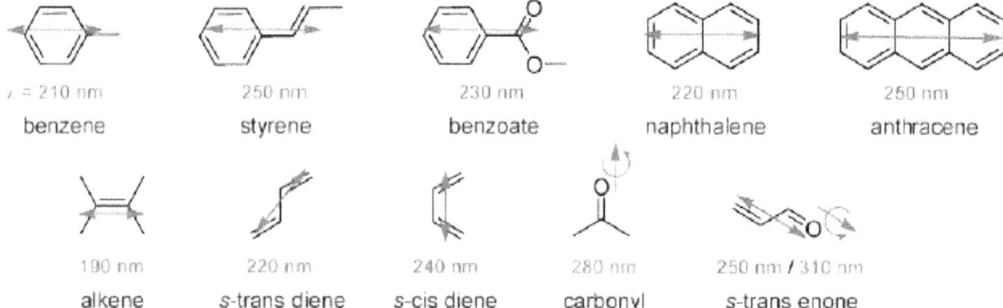

Fig. 2: Example for chromophores and their absorption wave length

Absorption of high energetic photon by the sample results in electronic transition from ground state to higher electronic states due to **molecular vibrations and electronic transitions (Fig. 3)** within the samples, which in turn causes modulation in the structure and environment of the chromophores, since the spectroscopy is also called as **electronic spectroscopy**.

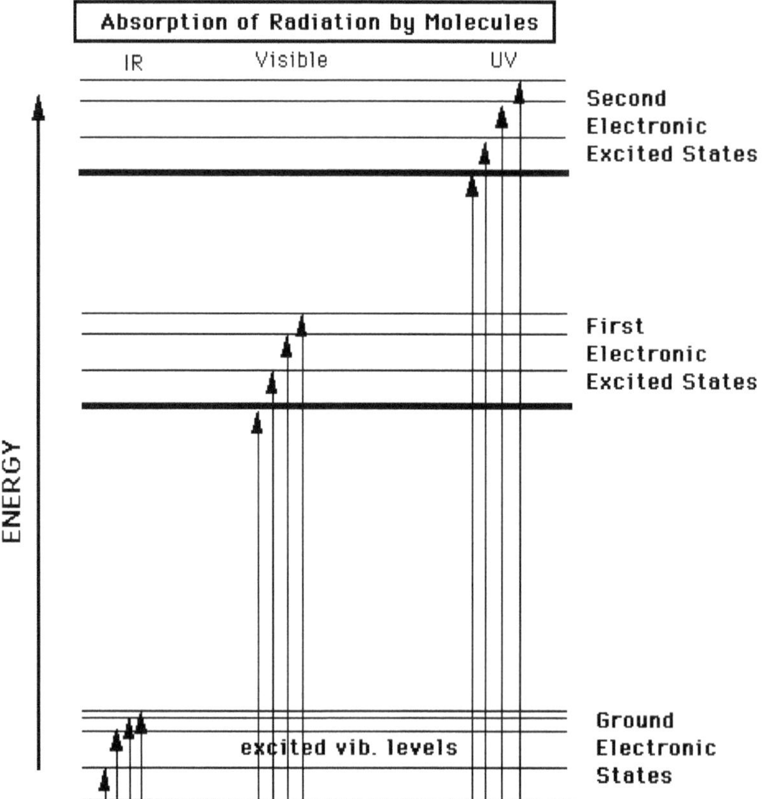

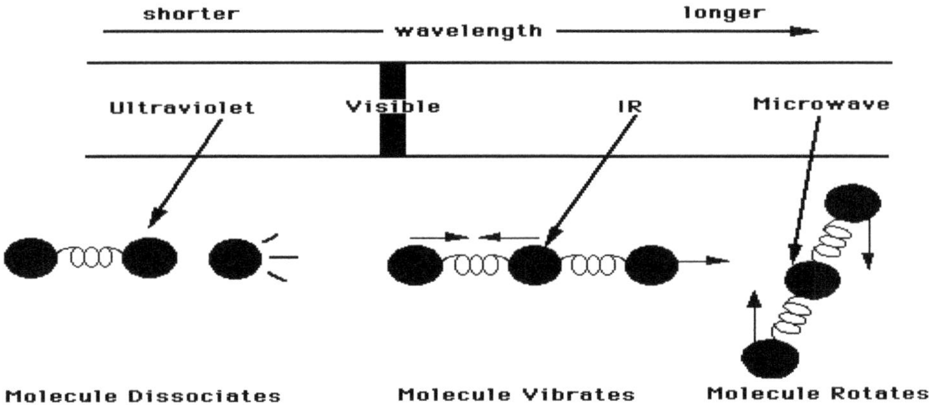

Fig. 3: Absorption of microwave causes rotation, IR causes vibration and UV causes transition of electrons in the sample

Missing of intensities at specific wavelength/frequency provides us the information on the chemical nature and environment of the sample represented as **spectra (Fig.4)**.

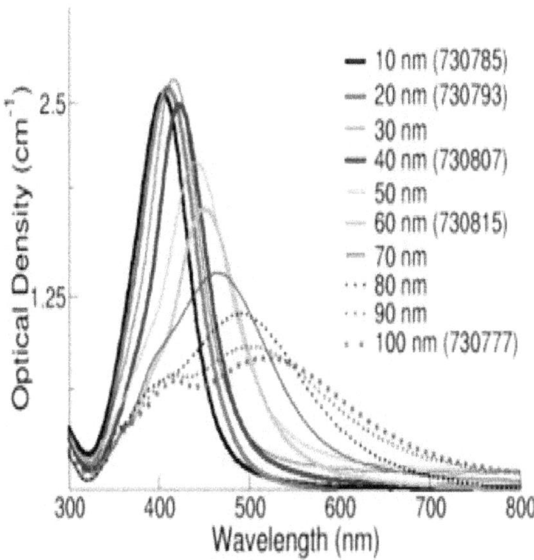

Fig. 4: Representation of UV spectra of silver nanoparticles at different concentration by observing wavelength (nm) in X-axis and Optical density ($Cm^{-1)}$ in Y-axis.

Principle of Operation

Beer-Lambert law: The quantity of light absorbed solution is directly proportional to the concentration of the substance and the path length of the light through the solution.

$$A = \log_{10} \frac{I_o}{I} = \varepsilon lc$$

A=Absorption of incident light
ε = Molar Absorptivity
l = Path length of the light
c = Concentration of the sample
I_o = Intensity of light entering the sample
I = Intensity of light emerging out of the sample

Construction of UV-Vis Spectroscopy

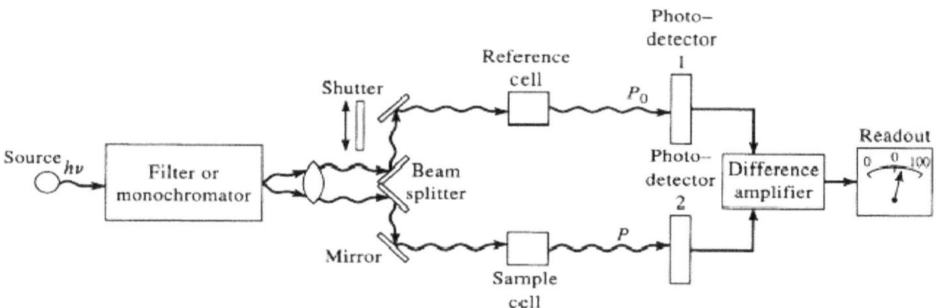

Components of UV-Vis Spectrometer

Light Source	:	Deuterium lamps and Tungsten filament lamps are the source of UV(160nm~375nm) and Visible light (400-700nm), respectively.
Shutter	:	Device that allows light to pass for a determined period.
Monochromator	:	Used as a filter to select a narrow portion of the spectrum of a given source.
Beam Splitter	:	A beam splitter is an optical device which can split an inciden light beam into two or more beams.
Cuvettes	:	A straight-sided clear container for holding liquid samples in a spectrophotometer. They may be made up of plastic, glass and quartz.
Detector	:	Used to detect the absorbed or transmitted light from the sample.Photovoltaic, Phototube and photo multiplier are the different detectors available at different generation of development.
Differential amplifier	:	Electronic amplifier that amplifies the difference between two input voltages but suppresses any voltage common to the two inputs
Recorder	:	A device that records and stores the data for future analysis.

Working Principle

Ultra violet and visible light are emitted from the respective sources are allowed to pass through monochromator to filter the unnecessary light of different wavelength. Light is allowed to fall on the biconvex lens and to beam splitter. Light from lens to beam splitter is controlled through an shutter. Here the beam is split in to two different path and directed to the sample and reference cell through a mirror. Reference cell consist of buffer or solvent alone whereas, sample cell contains active molecule in buffer or solvent. When the light encounters the sample cell, the active molecules present in the sample cell will absorb some wavelength of light from the incident light and falls on differential amplifier. Whereas, light passing through the reference cell which is devoid of active molecules suffers less absorption and falls on a differential amplifier. Differential amplifier amplifies the difference between two input voltages but suppresses any voltage common to the two inputs and displayed as a spectra with wavelength in X axis and optical density in Y axis. Results are recorded using a recorder for further analysis of spectra in future. The missing of intensities at specific wavelength/frequency provides us the information on the chemical nature and environment of the sample.

Application

a) Detection of impurities
b) Structure elucidation of organic compounds
c) Quantitative analysis of compounds
d) Chemical kinetics
e) Detection of functional group
f) Molecular weight determination
g) Estimation of concentration of sample.

Advantage

Due to, quick analysis takes less time and easy operating procedure it is widely used in all the field of research

Disadvantage

a) Scattering of light due to particulate in the sample
b) Cannot be used in higher concentration of the sample.
c) Stray light

11

Fourier Transform Infra Red (FTIR) Spectroscopy

Dr. Pon. Sathya Moorthy

A narrow spectrum of infrared (IR) spectrum lies between **visible light and microwave radiation.** Typical infrared spectrum covers between **2.5 μm to 25 μm** (2500 nm to 25000 nm) **or 400-4000 cm-1.** Infrared spectroscopy is one of the most important analytical technique in the field of advanced science. Infrared spectroscopy is a technique based on the **vibrations of the atoms** of a molecule. The molecule must possess a specific feature, i.e. an **electric dipole moment** which changes during the application of IR radiation. The dipole moment of an **IR active, heteronuclear diatomic** molecule changes its bond by **stretching and bending**. Whereas, **infrared-inactive' molecule is a homonuclear diatomic molecule** because its dipole moment remains zero no matter how long the bond. The interactions of infrared radiation with matter may be understood in terms of **changes in molecular dipoles associated with vibrations and rotations.** Liquids, solutions, pastes, powders, films, fibers, gases and surfaces which posses **electric dipole moment** can be examined through this technique. **IR active molecules** have unique IR absorption spectra that may be used as a "**fingerprint**" for identification.

Schematic Representation of FTIR Spectrometer

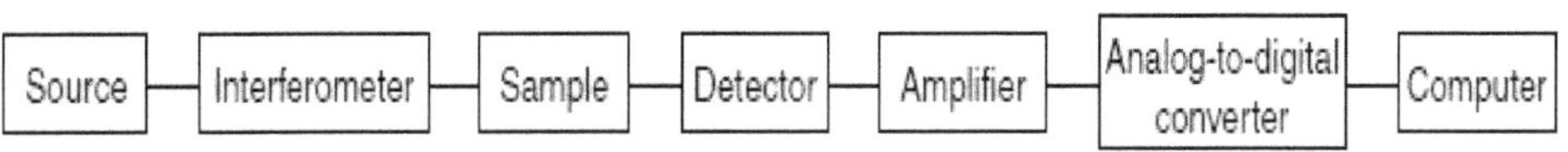

Source	:	Incandescent lamps are used in FTIR spectroscopy
Interferometer	:	An instrument in which the interference of two beams of light is employed to make precise measurements. It is the heart of the instrument (Fig. 1)
Sample holder	:	An experimental setup where the samples are place to characterize.

Detector	:	Used to detect the absorbed or transmitted light from the sample.
Amplifier	:	Amplifier is an electronic device that can increase the power of a signal
ADC	:	Analog to digital converter is an electronic system which converts an analog signal, into a digital signal.
Recorder	:	A device that records and stores the data for future analysis

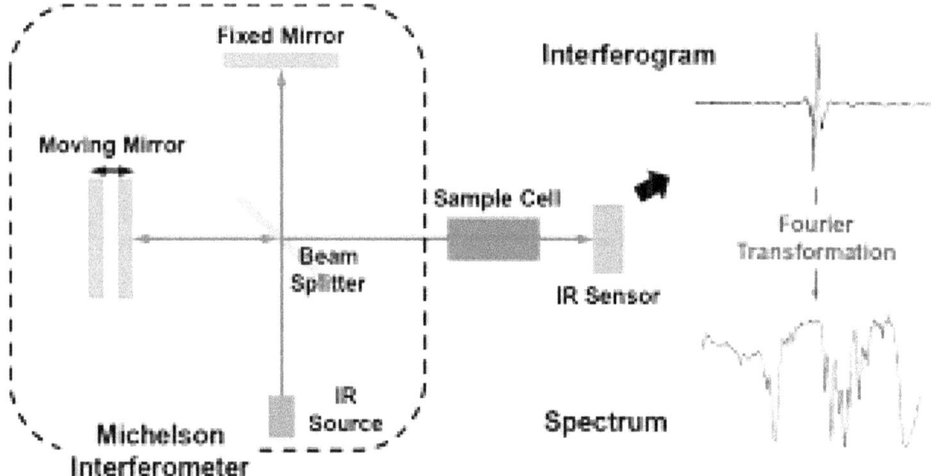

Fig. 1: Schematic representation of an Interferometer

Working Principle

Light is emitted from the source will travel in straight line and encounters a beam splitter. Beam splitter splits the beam in to two and allows to travel equal in horizontal and vertical direction as shown in the Fig.1. The light which travels in horizontal direction will fall on a movable mirror (which may travels either towards or away from the beam splitter) and reflected back to beam splitter. Whereas, the light travels in a vertical direction falls on a fixed mirror and reflected back to beam splitter. It's understood that the path traced by the light in horizon path may be short or longer than the light travelled in vertical direction which causes path difference between the two waves. The reflected light in vertical and horizontal direction falls back on the beam splitter causes superposition of waves. The superposed light produced **is a function of the change of path length** between the two beams. The superposed light is allowed to fall on a sample holder containing reference molecule (KBr pellet) having zero absorbance value is detected and stored. Now the KBr with our sample of interest is placed in the sample cell and absorption are detected and stored. The difference between a reference spectrum (no sample, KBr alone) and a sample spectrum (with sample, KBr with active morecule) gives us the IR absorption spectrum. The **"missing" intensities"** at specific energies give us the information on the vibrational properties of the sample. Amplifier, amplifies the signal, in which **high-frequency contributions** have been **eliminated by a filter**, the data are converted to digital form by an **analog-to-digital converter** and transferred to the computer for Fourier-transformation. The collected **absorption signals (or) interferograms are then converted into spectra** (Fig. 2. wavenumber *vs*. transmission plots) using a computer software).

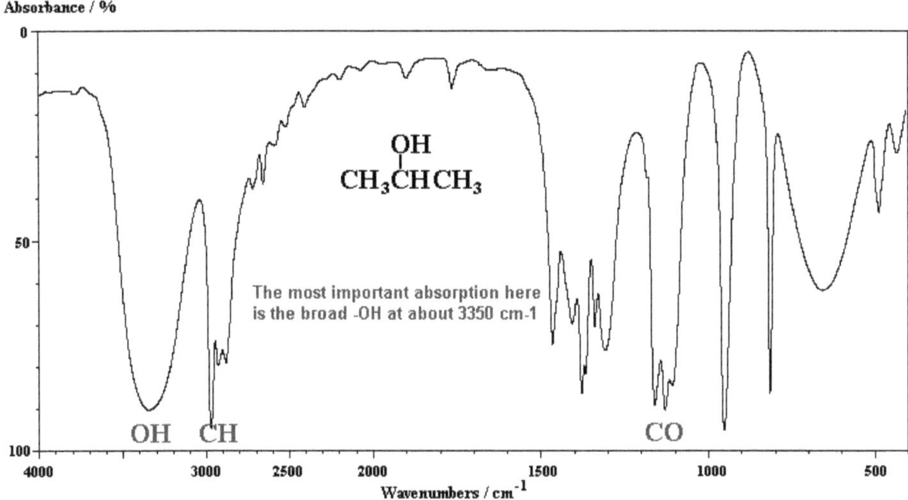

Fig. 2: FTIR spectra for a Propanol (C_3H_7OH) depicting the absorbance at 3400 cm-1 for OH 3000 cm^{-1} for CH and 1100 cm^{-1} for CO

Applications

FT-IR spectroscopy used to....

a) Identification of polymers and polymer blends.

b) Indirect verification of trace organic contaminants on surfaces.

c) Routine qualitative & quantitative FTIR Analysis.

d) Thin film analysis.

e) Analysis of adhesives, coatings and adhesion promoters or coupling agents.

f) Small visible particle chemical analysis.

g) Analysis of stains and surface blemishes remnant from cleaning and degreasing processes combined with optical microscopy.

h) Analysis of resins, composite materials and release films.

i) Solvent extractions of leachable or contaminants, plasticisers, mould release agents and weak boundary layers coupled with XPS surface chemical analysis techniques.

j) Identification of rubbers and filled rubbers.

k) Determination of degrees of crystallinity in polymers. Comparative chain lengths in organics.

l) Measure air pollutants

m) Monitoring heavy metal from wastewater

Advantages

a) Feglet or multiplex advantage arises because all spectral elements are measured simultaneously, so the spectrum can be obtained quickly.

b) Jacquinet ot throughput advantage arise due to the absence of slits which attenuates the IR light. So the optical throughput of the spectrometer is enhanced

c) Connes advantage arise due to the frequency scale of spectrum is known accurately.

d) All the above advantages reduce the signal to noise ratio of the spectra.

Disadvantages

a) FTIR instrument do not measure the spectra directly computer for transforming interferogram to spectra.

b) FTIR cannot be used for **homonuclear diatomic molecules.**

Self-assessment Questions

1. ______________ lies between visible light and microwave radiation
2. Typical infrared spectrum covers between ______________.
3. diatomic molecule are IR active molecules.
4. ______________ diatomic molecules are IR inactive molecules.
5. Unique IR absorption spectra that may be used as a ______________ for identification.
6. ______________ is an IR inactive molecule.
7. ______________ is the heart of FTIR spectrometer.
8. Two equal opposite charges separated by a distance is called as ___________
9. ______________ advantages increase the SNR of the spectra.
10. 10. Incandescent lamps are used as a source in FTIR spectroscopy: **True or False.**

For further reading

Fundamentals of UV-Vis Spectroscopy by Tony Owen, Hewlett-Packard publication number 12-5965-5123E. 1996.

UV-VIS Spectroscopy and Its Applications by Heinz-Helmut Perkampus, Springer-Verlag Berlin Heidelberg, 1992.

12

Structural Characterization of Nanomaterials Using X-ray Diffraction Technique

Dr S Marimuthu

The discovery of X-rays by Wilhelm Conrad Roentgen, the first Nobel laureate in physics, in 1895 and later, Max von Laue's experiment on the diffraction of crystals for X rays, gave a powerful tool for the investigation of crystal structure. X-rays are electromagnetic radiation with typical photon energies in the range of 100 eV - 100 keV. Short wavelength x-rays (hard x-rays) in the range of a few angstroms to 0.1 angstrom (1 keV - 120 keV) are used for diffraction applications. X-rays have wavelengths from ~0.1 to ~100 Å, which are located between γ -radiation and ultraviolet rays. The wavelengths, ranged between ~0.5 and ~2.5 Å are used in diffraction studies, since the wavelength of X-rays is comparable to the size of atoms, are ideally suited for studying structural arrangement of atoms and molecules in materials.

About 95 per cent of solid materials are crystalline in nature, where atoms are arranged with symmetric repeats. When X-rays interact with a crystalline substance, it results in characteristic diffraction pattern. The same substance always gives the same pattern; and in a mixture of substances, each produces its pattern independently of others. The X-ray diffraction pattern of particular substance is like a fingerprint of the substance, which helps to identify the unknown substances. Similarly, X-ray diffraction is also useful in determination of phase of the materials, crystallite size and lattice stresses

To summarize, X-ray diffraction is an analytical technique looking at X-ray scattering from crystalline materials. Each material produces a unique X-ray "fingerprint" of X-ray intensity versus scattering angle that is characteristic of its crystalline atomic structure.

How X-rays are Produced

X-rays are produced from X- ray tube it is a device, which consists of cathode and anode. The cathode acts as the source of electrons, which are accelerated to strike the anode (Grounded) and the cathode, is maintained at a high negative potential with respect to the anode. The anode acts as source of producing X-rays (Fig 1). The high voltage maintained across cathode and anode, some tens of thousands of volts, rapidly draws the electrons to the anode, which they strike with very high velocity. X-rays are produced at the point of impact over anode and radiate in all directions.

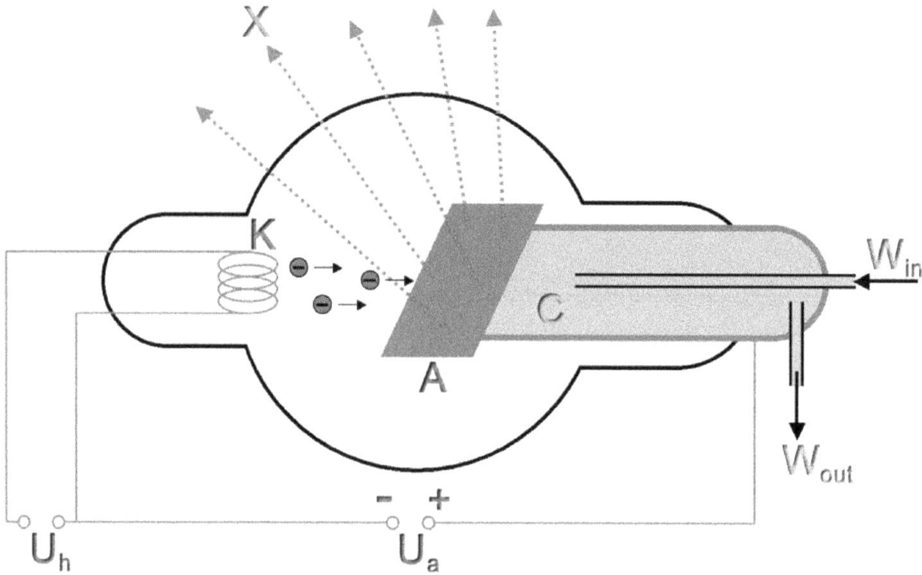

Fig. 1: X-ray tube consists of K (cathode) and A (anode mostly metal targets) biased with positive potential. C refers to chiller unit for dissipating heat from anodes and X are X- rays

When the target material of the X-ray tube is bombarded with fast moving electrons from the cathode filament, two types of X-ray spectra are produced, which are continuous and characteristic X-rays. When electrons from cathode interact in the vicinity of target nucleus of an atom, it results in *Bremsstrahlung* production caused by the deceleration and change in momentum of incident electrons. This process causes continuous production of X-rays with less intensity which continues as long as the applied voltage in the X-ray tube is insufficient to remove electrons near the nucleus in K shell (Fig 2). Generally, the intensity of continuous X-ray is directly proportional to the voltage applied in the X-ray tube, beam current and atomic number of metal target. When the incident electron has greater energy than the K-shell binding energy, it ejects electron in K shell creating vacancy. The electrons from outer shells transit to inner vacancy emitting X-rays with energy equal to the difference in binding energies of outer shells and K-shell during the transition.

The X-rays are referred as characteristic radiation of anode materials used in the X- ray tube. When an electron falls from the L- shell to the K shell, the X-ray is referred as K-alpha X-ray, while an electron transits from M-shell to K-shell,

X-ray is called a K-beta X-rays. Kα X-rays have higher intensity than Kβ X-rays. Kα X-rays are used in the X-ray diffraction technique. The characteristic X-rays are monochromatic in nature and frequency of emission depends on the anode materials. Copper is the most common target material in X-ray diffraction technique with wavelength of CuKα radiation = 1.54184 Å.

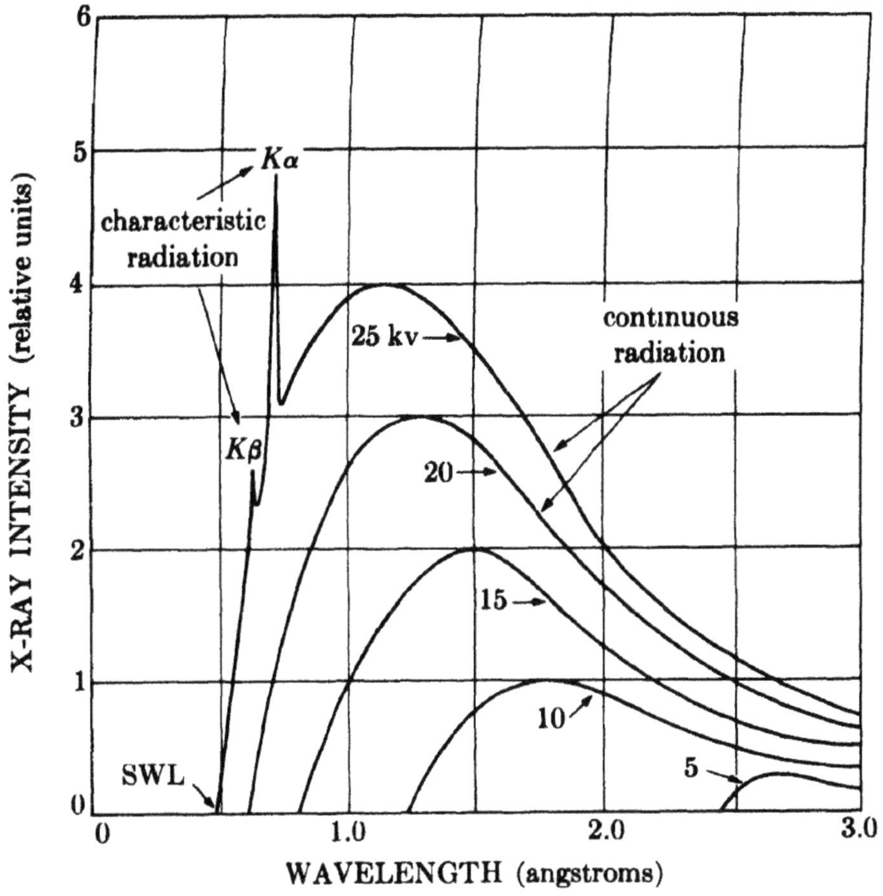

(Adopted from Elements of X-ray Diffraction by B D Cullity)

Fig 2: Continuous radiation or Bremsstrahlung spectra produced initially with low voltage, and the characteristic X-ray radiation is monochromatic in nature with high intensity (Kα and Kβ)

Braggs' Law

When an X-ray beam hits an atom in the sample, the electrons around the atom start to oscillate with the same frequency as the incoming radiation. When the diffracted waves are out of phase, destructive interference takes place resulting no radiant energy leaving the sample. However if atoms in a crystal are arranged in a regular pattern, the resultant diffracting waves on interaction will have constructive interference in a very few directions (Fig 3). The constructive interference results in sharp interference maxima (peaks) with the same symmetry as in the distribution of atoms. Measuring the diffraction pattern therefore allows deducing the distribution of atoms in a material and the peaks in a X-ray diffraction pattern are directly related to the atomic distances.

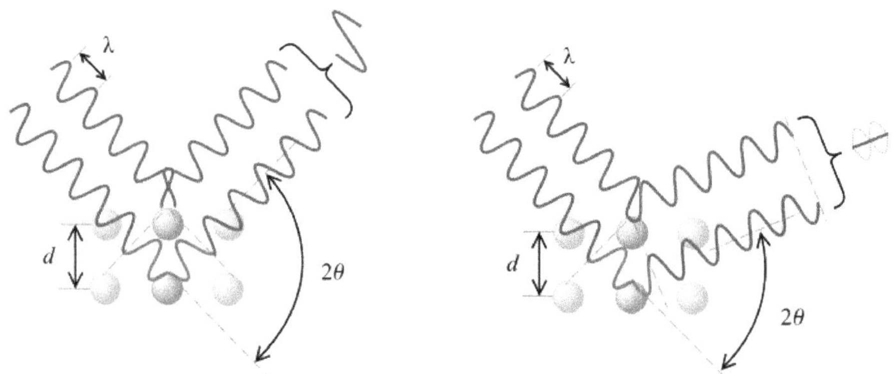

Fig 3: Constructive Interference (left) takes place when diffracted waves are in phase and destructive interference takes place (right) when diffracted waves are out of phase

The fundamental law, which governs the x-ray diffraction phenomenon, is the Bragg's Law, which relates the wavelength of electromagnetic radiation to the diffraction angle and the lattice spacing (interatomic spacing) in a crystalline sample, when the interaction of the incident rays with the sample produces constructive interference. Bragg's Law refers to the simple equation,

$$n\lambda = 2d \operatorname{Sin} \theta$$

The equations was derived mathematically by the English physicists Sir W.H. Bragg and his son Sir W.L. Bragg in 1913 to explain the reflection of X ray beams at certain angles of incidence (theta, theta) from the cleavage faces of crystals. The variable *d* is the distance between atomic layers in a crystal, and the variable lambda (**λ**) is the wavelength of the incident X-ray beam and n is an integer

Let us consider two X-ray beam incident on a pair of parallel planes L1 and L2, separated by an interatomic spacing d (Fig 4) The X-ray on plane L1 reflects back as θ as normal law of reflection and similarly X ray on plane L2 also reflected back with θ angle. However, the path length difference for X-ray fall on L2 is AB + BC

Since AB and AC are equal in distance, let us consider it as $a + a = 2a$

According to the trigonometry, $Sin\Theta = a/d$ or $a = d\ Sin\ \theta$

or $2a = 2dSin\ \theta$ or $n\lambda = 2dSin\ \theta$

Hence, reflected beam will result maximum intensity, if the waves are in phase. The difference in path length between the waves must be an integral number of wavelengths as follows Braggs' law.

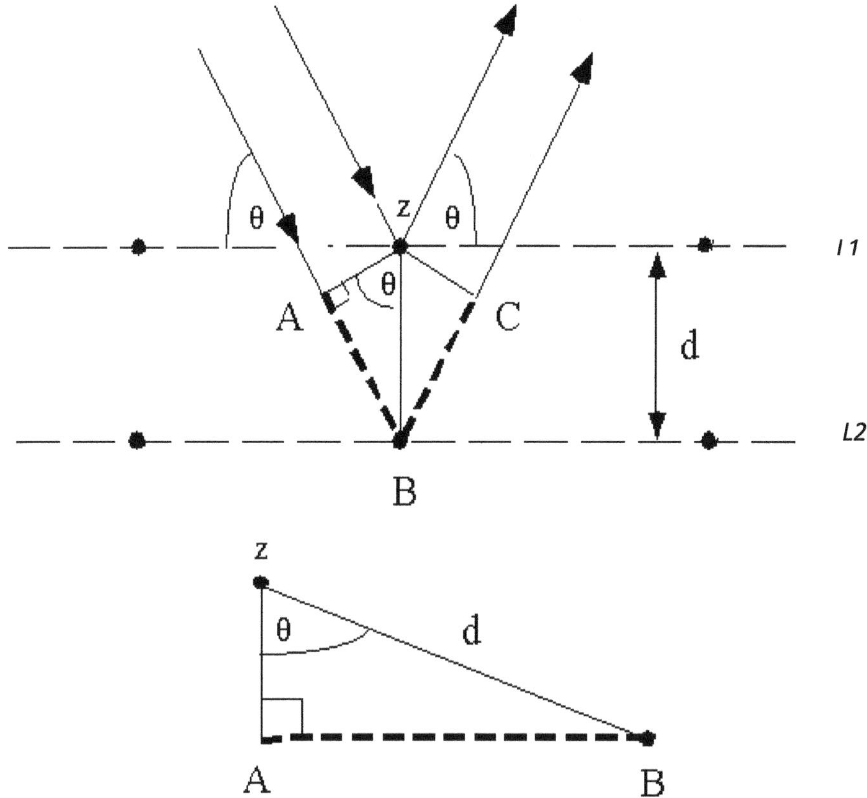

Fig. 4: Derivation of Braggs' law when the diffracted beam interfere constructively

X-ray Diffractometer

X-ray diffraction is based on constructive interference of monochromatic X-rays and a crystalline sample. A cathode ray tube, filtered to produce monochromatic radiation, collimated to concentrate, and directed toward the sample, generates X-rays. The interaction of the incident rays with the sample produces constructive interference (and a diffracted ray) when conditions satisfy Bragg's Law ($n\lambda=2d \sin \theta$). The diffracted X-rays are then detected, processed and counted. All possible diffraction directions of the lattice in the sample are attained by scanning the sample through a range of 2Θ angles. Conversion of the diffraction peaks to d spacing allows identification of the mineral because each mineral has a set of unique d spacing

The instrument used for X-ray diffraction studies is X-ray diffractometer, which consist of three basic components, an X-ray tube; a sample holder, and an X-ray detector. X-rays are generated in a cathode ray tube (Tungsten) by heating a filament to produce electrons, which are accelerated to impinge a target (metal node. Normally copper) by applying very high voltage. Cobalt and Molybdenum are used as anodes in X-ray diffraction technique. When electrons have sufficient energy to dislodge inner shell K electrons of the target metal and characteristic X-rays are produced. Crystal monochrometers are required to produce monochromatic X-rays needed for diffraction. The fine-grained powder under investigation are placed at the designated place in glass plate. Gentle pressing flattens the sample and avoids air pockets in the sample. The glass plate along with sample are kept in the sample holder. The X-rays are collimated and directed onto the sample.

The geometry of an X-ray diffractometer is such that the x ray tube rotates in the path of the collimated X-ray beam at an angle θ while the X-ray detector, mounted on an arm to collect the diffracted X-rays, rotates at an angle of 2θ, which is known as Bragg-Brentano configuration. The mechanism used to maintain the angle and rotate the X-ray tube and detector is termed as Goniometer (Fig 5). The intensity of diffracted X- rays is continuously recorded as the sample and detector rotate through respective angles normally from 5° to 90°. When the geometry of the incident X-rays impinging the sample satisfies the Braggs' equation, constructive interference occurs results in peak intensity (maxima in the spectra). The diffracted X-rays are then detected, processed and counted

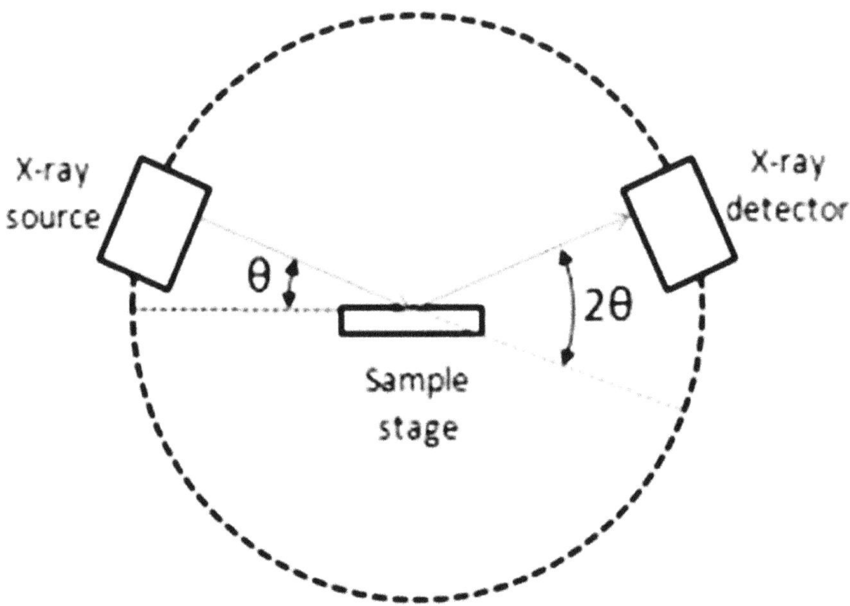

Fig. 5: The main components of X-ray diffractometer are X-ray tube, sample stage and X ray detector. The Goniometer keeps x ray tube at angle θ while keeping the arm of the detector at 2θ

After a scan of the sample the X-ray intensity are plotted against the angle θ to produce a chart showing diffraction peak corresponding the angle 2θ which are converted to d spacing, using the Bragg equation. Conversion of the diffraction peaks to d spacing allows identification of the sample under investigation because each mineral has a set of unique d spacing. The comparison of spectra from the sample are compared with standard reference patterns of International Centre for Crystal Diffraction (ICCD) who have collected data diffraction peak and 2θ for thousands of crystalline substances for identifying the sample.

Applications

- X-ray diffraction has widespread applications in the fields of geology, pharmaceuticals, materials, polymers, environmental and forensic investigations
- Identification of unknown crystalline substances and determination of crystallite size
- Measurement of strain, or micro-strain effects (imperfections) in bulk and thin-film samples
- Quantification of preferred orientation (texture) in thin films, multi-layer stacks, and manufactured parts
- Determination of the ratio of crystalline to amorphous material in bulk materials and thin-film samples
- Analyzing films as thin as 50 angstroms for texture and phase behaviors
- Determining strain and composition in epitaxial thin films and, surface offcut in single crystal materials
- Measuring residual stress in bulk metals and ceramics

Advantages

- X-ray diffraction is a non-destructive technique
- Reliable and powerful tool for the identification of crystalline minerals
- Simple sample preparation
- X-ray diffraction is faster method and deriving results are simple and straight forward

Limitations

- X-ray diffraction is highly suitable for identifying single phase material
- Standard library is essential for interpreting results
- X-ray diffraction requires sample grain size of 2μ
- Detection limit for phase identification in the sample is ~ 2 to 5 per cent.
- Identification of amorphous materials is difficult through X ray diffraction

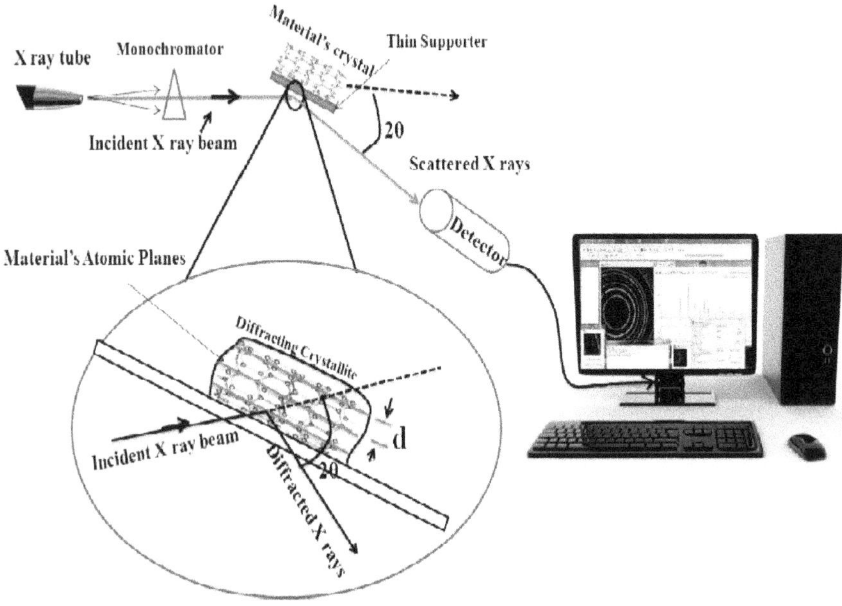

Fig. 6: Schematic illustration of X-ray Diffractometer (Adopted from Das *et al.*, 2014)

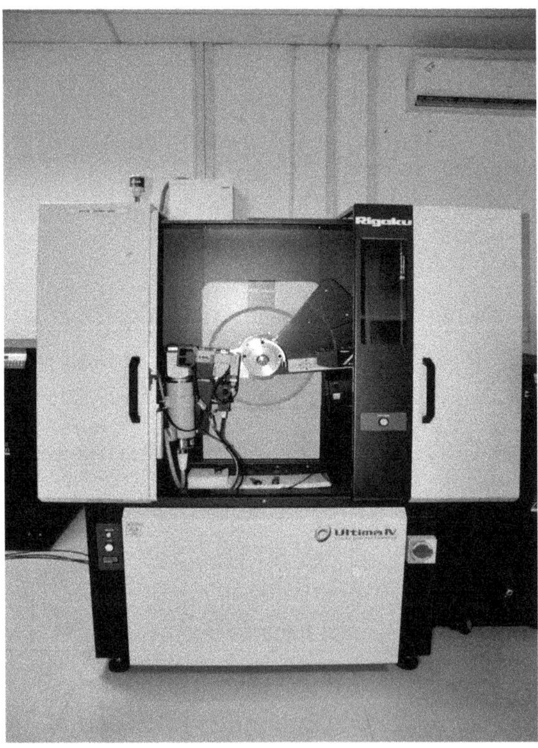

Fig. 7: X-ray Diffractometer (Rigaku Model Ultima IV)

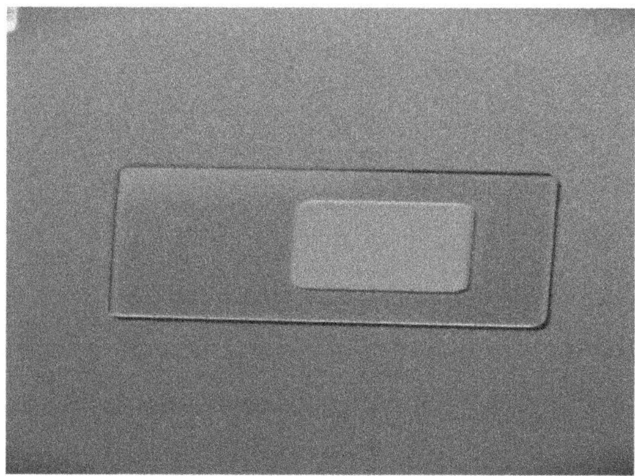

Fig. 8: Glass plate sample holder with designated area (depression) for filling sample

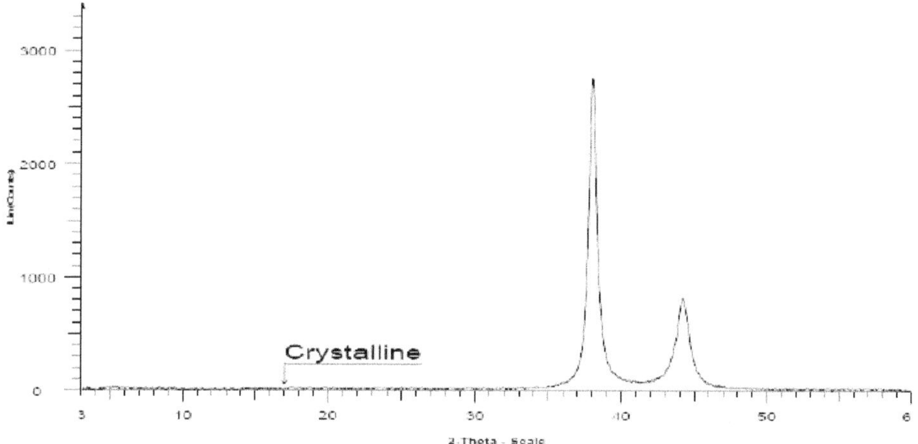

Fig. 9: X-ray diffraction pattern of crystalline sample with sharp intense peaks

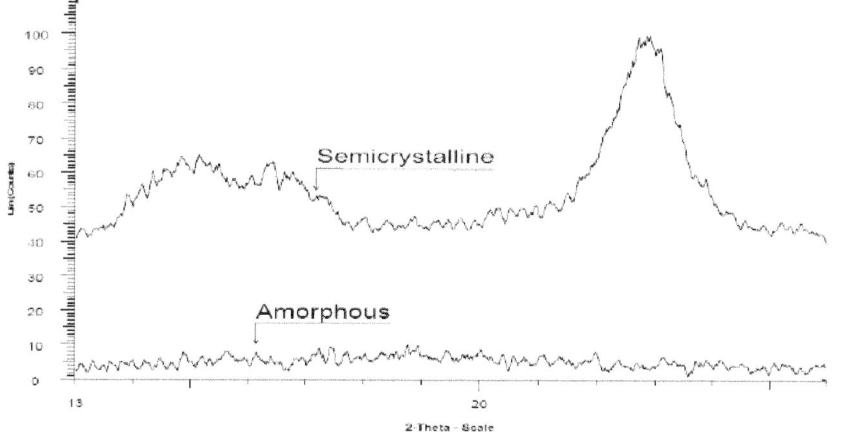

Fig. 10: X-ray diffraction pattern of semi crystalline and amorphous samples

Self-assessment Questions

1. Define Braggs' law
2. Define Goniometer
3. Illustrate X-ray Diffractometer
4. Expand ICDD
5. Differentiate continuous and characteristic X-rays
6. Describe the instrumentation of X-ray Diffraction with illustration
7. Describe the working principle and instrumentation of X-ray Diffraction
8. List out the applications of X-ray Diffraction technique
9. Write the advantages and limitation of X-ray Diffraction technique
10. How X-rays are produced in X-ray diffractometer?

Fill in the blanks

1. ____________________ discovered X-rays
2. ____________________ cathode used for generating electrons
3. ____________________, anode used for producing X-rays
4. ________________ maintains X-ray tube at θ and X-ray detector at 2θ angles
5. The diffracted rays follows Braggs' equation when they interfere________
6. ________ and __________ are father and son who received Noble Prize in physics.

13

Biosensor: Principles and Applications in Agriculture

Dr M. Djanaguiraman

Genesis and Background

The word "sensor" find its origin from the Latin word "sentire" which basically means 'to identify' anything. By hearing the word sensor, the primary thing that spirals into our minds is the concept of basic five human senses. The working mechanism of these senses is a) reception of input signal by the sensory cells due to external stimuli, b) conduction of signal towards the brain for interpretation as neurological impulses, and c) receptors respond to the stimulus as per instructed by the interoperating center. The genesis of sensor has started long time ago; people have used indications like weight of a fish in a pond or its viability and color change in leaves as a potential water and soil contaminants. In 19th century canaries have been used in coal mining as an early warning system to indicate the release of poisonous gases like carbon monoxide, methane and other gases accumulated in coal mines. Human nose and tongue are very sensitive to nature, which can tell us about content and nature of the chemical or material. One of the best known sensor is the litmus paper test for acids and alkalis, which provides a qualitative indication by means of colour reaction. Similarly, pH meter is also a type of sensor.

Griffin and Nelson have demonstrated for the first time immobilization of invertase enzyme on aluminium hydroxide or charcoal and the enzyme bound to insoluble support retains its activity. This is the milestone in the development of biosensor. However, the first true biosensor was developed by Leland C. Clark, Jr in 1956 for oxygen detection. He is known as the father of biosensors and his invention of the oxygen electrode bears his name Clark electrode. The Clark oxygen electrode laid the basis for the first glucose biosensor, followed by sensor for detection of urea. In 1975, the first commercial biosensor for analyzing whole blood glucose level was developed by Yellow Spring Instruments, Ohio, USA. From the time when the development of the i-STAT sensor, *i.e.*, portable clinical analyzer or point of care analyzer, tremendous progress have been observed in the field of biosensor. Biosensor is a cross cutting field involving physics, chemistry and biology with fundamentals of biology, nanotechnology and electronics.

A sensor is a device which receives and responds to a signal or stimulus. A biosensor is an analytical device containing a biological recognition element like immobilized enzyme, antibody, nucleic acid, hormone, organelle or whole cell, which can specially interact with the analyte of interest and produce physical, chemical or electrical signals that can be measured. Technically speaking, biosensing is a phenomenon that reserves set techniques for the production of an accessible detection signal by the interaction of biological molecules with an output device.

Features of Ideal Biosensor

- Reproducibility is the ability of the biosensor to generate identical responses for a duplicated experimental set-up.
- Stability is the degree of susceptibility to ambient disturbances in and around the biosensing system.
- Accuracy or precision: The biosensors should provide acceptable accuracy (±5%) and precision over relevant ranges of analyte measurement.
- Selectivity is the ability of a bioreceptor to detect a specific analyte in a sample containing other admixtures and contaminants.
- Sensitivity: The minimum amount of analyte that can be detected by a biosensor defines its limit of detection (LOD) or sensitivity. This usually needs to be sub-millimolar, but in special cases can go down to the femtomolar (10^{-15} M) range.
- Linearity is the attribute that shows the accuracy of the measured response. Mathematically it is represented as y=mc, where y is the output signal, m is the sensitivity of the biosensor and c is the concentration of the analyte. Linearity of the biosensor can be associated with the resolution of the biosensor and range of analyte concentrations under test.
- Times: (i) The response time is usually much longer than with chemical sensors. It may be 30 s or longer, (ii) The recovery time is the time before a biosensor is ready to analyze the next sample. It must not be too long i.e., not more than a few minutes, (iii) the working lifetime is usually determined by the instability of the biological material. It can vary from a few days to a few months.
- Simplicity: Lower cost, and less likely to be incorrectly made.
- Continuous: In some cases, the close monitoring of analyte levels over time may be critical. In that case the biosensor should be continuous.

Components of Biosensor

A biosensor mainly consists of two parts, (i) biological component for sensing the presence and concentration of a analyte (substance to be determined), which constitutes enzyme, antibodies etc. and (ii) a transducer device, which collects information from the biological component, converts, amplifies and display them. The various components of biosensor are presented in Fig. 1. In order to form a biosensor, the biological particles are immobilized on the transducer surface which acts as a point of contact between the transducer and analyte. When a biosensor is used to analyze a sample for an analyte of interest, the biological part specific to the analyte molecules, interacts specifically and efficiently leading to production of a physicochemical change on the transducer surface. This change is picked up by the transducer and gets converted into any measurable signals. The produced signal undergoes amplification, interpretation and finally display signals accounting to the amount of analyte present in the sample.

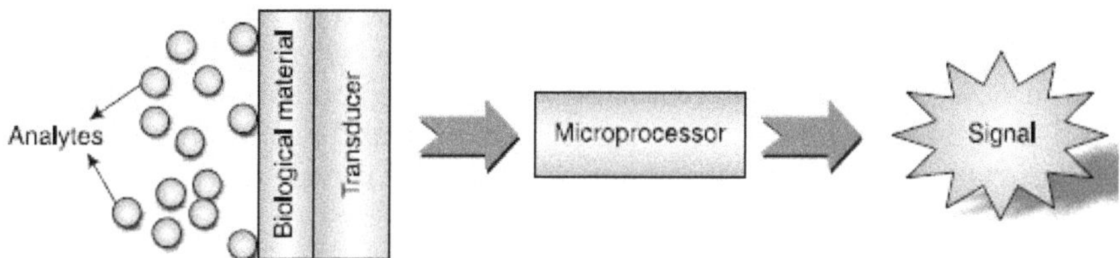

Fig. 1. The main components of a biosensor (Long *et al.*, 2013; Sensors 13:13928-13948)

Classification of Biosensor

Based on Activity

Biosensor can be classified into two types namely catalytic (metabolism) and non-catalytic (affinity) biosensor. The non-catalytic biosensor is classified into two types namely labelled affinity sensor and non-labelled affinity sensor. Enzyme electrode is an example for catalytic or kinetic biosensor. Enzyme labelled, fluorescence and immunosensor are the examples for labeled affinity sensor. Surface plasmon resonance and piezoelectric are the examples for label free affinity sensor.

Based on Analyte

Based on analyte, biosensor can be classified into four types namely enzyme, DNA, immuno and microbial biosensor, if the analyte was enzyme, DNA, antibody and microbes, respectively.

Based on Biological Receptor

Bioreceptor can be of three types namely (i) biological materials: e.g. tissue, microorganisms, organelles, cell receptors, enzymes, antibodies, nucleic acids, natural products etc., (ii) biologically derived materials: e.g. recombinant antibodies, engineered proteins, aptamers etc. and (iii) biomimics: e.g. synthetic receptors, biomimetic catalysts, combinatorial ligands, imprinted polymers etc.

Based on Detection mode or Transducer or Signal Transduction Principles

Four basic types of transducers namely electrochemical, optical, piezoelectric and thermal transducers are used for the construction of biosensors. The mode of action of transducer is presented in table 1.

Table 1. Principle and mode of action and applications of various transducer

Sl. No.	Transducer system	Principle
1.	Electrochemical	Change in electric signal
2.	Optical	Change in absorbance or fluorescence
3.	Piezoelectric	Change in mass
4.	Thermal	Change in temperature

Electrochemical: There are three basic electrochemical process which are used in transducer. (i) potentiometry, the measurement of a cell potential at zero current; (ii) amperometry, in which an oxidising (or reducing) potential is applied between the cell electrodes and the cell current is measured; and (iii) conductimetry, where the conductance (reciprocal of resistance) of the cell is measured by an alternating current bridge method.

Optical transducer: In optical transducer chemical energy is converted to light energy. Optical transduction utilizes the changes in optical properties like phase, amplitude, and frequency established because of the selective binding of an analyte with the bioreceptors. In colorimetric change in light adsorbed as reactant are converted to products is measured. In photometric, photon output for a luminescent or fluorescent process can be detected with a photomultiplier tubes or photodiode systems.

Piezoelectric devices: involve the generation of electric currents from a vibrating crystal. The frequency of vibration is affected by the mass of material adsorbed on its surface, which could be related to an active biochemical reaction. Microscale cantilever beams can also be used to identify the mass of the biomolecules upon interaction with a specific biomolecule. The level of deflection by cantilever beam can be measured which indicates the amount of analyte in the solution.

Thermal methods: A temperature transducer is a device that converts the thermal quantity into any physical quantity namely mechanical energy, pressure and electrical signals etc. The best example is thermocouple, in which the electrical potential difference is produced due to temperature difference across its terminals. Hence, thermocouple is a temperature transducer. Similarly, thermistors are semiconductor devices which behave as thermal resistors having a high negative temperature coefficient of resistance. There are two types of thermistors (negative temperature coefficient and positive temperature coefficient) are available in market. All chemical and biochemical processes involve the production or absorption of heat. This heat can be measured by sensitive thermistors and hence be related to the amount of reaction.

Biorecognition Elements

The biosensor available today has five major bioreceptor for signal recognition namely (i) enzymes, (ii) antibodies, (iii) protein/peptide receptors, (iv) nucleic acids and (v) whole cell receptors, which are explained in detail below:

Enzyme

Enzymes are proteins, i.e., biopolymers that consist of α-amino acid residues connected by amide linkages and which exert catalytic activity. An enzyme usually containing a prosthetic group, which often has one or more metal atoms. The enzymes used in biosensor involves oxidation or reduction as mode of action which can be detected electrochemically. The application of various enzymes in the biosensor assembly is provided in table 2. Enzyme biosensor are specific to the substrate, their catalytic activity causes higher sensitivity and they consume less time. However, the cost of extracting, isolating and purifying enzyme is very high. Sometimes enzyme losses its activity when they are immobilized on a transducer. The enzyme may lose activity, owing to deactivation, after a relatively short period of time.

Antibodies

Antibodies are also known as immunoglobulins or g-globulins. It is Y-shaped serum glycoproteins that are produced as a response to foreign substances called antigens. Antibodies can be of three types polyclonal, monoclonal and recombinant antibodies. Antibodies are very specific, and some antibodies can distinguish the enantiomers of the same organic molecule. Both antibodies (Ab) and antigen (Ag) molecules can be detected using immunoassay (enzyme linked immunosorbent assay; ELISA) approaches, but more frequently the Ag molecules are considered as target. The enzyme-linked immunoassays can be linked with the electroanalytical methods namely ampherometric enzyme linked immunoassays, amperometric assays based on the Clarke oxygen electrode, amperometric immunoassays labelled with an electroactive species and potentiometric immunoassay.

Table 2. Application of various enzymes in the biosensor assembly

Enzyme name	Analyte	Application area
Glucose oxidase	Glucose	Health industry, food industry and biotechnology
Glucose-6-phosphate dehydrogenase	Glucose, phosphate	Environmental monitoring
Tyrosinase	Phenol	Environmental monitoring
Peroxidase	H_2O_2, phenols, aromatic amines	Auxiliary enzyme for enzyme sensors based on other oxidoreductases, medicine, pharmaceutics and microbe industry, environmental monitoring
Urease	Urea	Fertilizer industry and heavy metal in soil

Acetylcholinesterase	Organophosphates, Carbamates	Pesticide residue
Tyrosinase/catechol	Triazines	Herbicide residue
Aldehyde dehydrogenase	Dithiocarbamates	Fungicide residue

Protein/Peptide Receptor

Synthetic peptides take intermediate place between the amino acids and proteins. The progress in the chemistry and application of synthetic peptides is related to high stability in extreme environment, high performance in organic solvents, and low cost. The peptide receptors showed increased affinity toward small organic molecules and hence it can be an alternative to antibodies analysis. The peptide based biorecognition assumes multi-point interaction with an analyte molecule that is based on non-covalent interactions, e.g., hydrogen bonding, the formation of salt bridges, and hydrophobic and van der Waals interactions. Regarding the application of peptides in biosensors, the signal transduction with peptide receptor is mainly based on the same principles as conventional immunoassay. The binding of specific analytes can be detected by changes in optical or electrical properties of the interface or by direct mass changes measured with QCM (Quartz Crystal Microbalance) technique.

Nucleic Acids

Nucleic acids bioreceptor works like antibodies in many ways. A DNA assay often involves the addition of labelled DNA to the assay. The labelling may be radioactive, photometric, enzymic or electroactive, giving scope for a range of biosensor types. In DNA sensors, short sequences (oligonucleotides) are used, many of them are selected from the polymerase chain reaction of the DNA amplification used in a traditional DNA assay for establishing particular sequences specific for hosting organisms. In analogy with the DNA assay techniques, such as oligonucleotide are also termed DNA probes. Contrary to the DNA probes, aptamers are fully synthetic oligonucleotides obtained *de novo* from the DNA (RNA) library by a combinatorial chemistry approach. A chemically synthesized library consists of 10^9-10^{15} molecules of the ss-DNA, each possessing a random-sequence region positioned between specific primer sequences for amplification.

Whole Cells

Whole cells can be used either in a viable or nonviable form. Viable cells can metabolize various organic compounds either anaerobically or aerobically resulting in various end products like ammonia, carbon dioxide, acids, and so forth that can be monitored using a variety of transducers. Cells have been often used because they have high sensitivity to adjacent environment. The attachment on the surface is the main characteristic of cells, so they can be easily immobilized. It is used to detect toxicity, organic derivatives and to monitor the treatment effects.

Application of Biosensor in Agricultural Sciences

Use of sensor and biosensor in medical science, environmental science, bioprocess control, quality control of food, biodefense and agriculture have been established. However, use of biosensor in medical science have grown to a great extent compared to agricultural science. Some of the potential applications of biosensor in agriculture are listed below:

Biosensor for Nitrogenous Compounds in Soil and Water

Urea is a nitrogen compound widely used as fertilizer in agriculture. The first urea potentiometric biosensor was built by urease immobilization on polyacrylamide gel on the surface of an ammonium ion-selective electrode. Potentiometry, optical, conductometry, colorimetry and amperometry transducing techniques were employed to detect urea. The nitrate form of nitrogen fertilizer is quantified using nitrate reductase enzyme based biosensor through amperometric technique. Nitrate can be quantified by cytochrome c nitrite reductase enzyme based on optical principle. Nitrate in water can be quantified using methyl viologen mediator mixed with nitrate reductase enzyme through conductimetric electrode.

Biosensor for Pesticide Residue in Soil and Water

Biosensors are designed to detect contaminants. Three main classes of pesticides that pose a serious problem are organophosphates, organochlorines and carbamates. Organophosphorus pesticides such as dichlorvos and paraoxon at very low levels can be monitored by liposome-based biosensor. Monitoring the level of pesticides in the environment typically employ the enzyme acetylcholinesterase. Furthermore, enzymes like cholinesterase, organophosphorus-hydrolase and urease are used in the design of electrochemical biosensors for pesticides detection. For the detection of herbicides such as phenyl urea and triazines, which inhibit photosynthesis, biosensors have been designed with membrane receptors of thylakoid and chloroplasts for which mainly amperometric and optical transductors is employed. The mechanism of detection, biorecognition element and analyte in pesticide detection was furnished in table 3.

Biosensor for Heavy Metals and Pollutant Detection in Soil and Water

Contaminates in soil is due to discharge of industrial effluents, which has significant amount of heavy metals. For example, many tannery industry areas are polluted with chromium because of discharge of tannery waste. Moreover, fertilizer has become one of the polluting sources of heavy metals. The majority of existing techniques used for trace analysis of heavy metals includes spectroscopic, voltammetric and chromatographic methods, which can detect species at low concentrations or even in single elements. For heavy metals detection, different enzymes such as acetylcholinesterase, alkaline phosphatase, urease, invertase, peroxidise, L-lactate dehydrogenase, tyrosinase, and nitrate reductase, have been used. The inhibition of the immobilized enzyme can be detected via electrochemical (amperometric, potentiometric, and conductometric) or optical measurements. The principle of detection and biorecognition element is resumed in Table 4. "Critters on a chip" consists of a tiny light-sensitive computer chip coated with bioluminescent bacteria. When the bacteria encounter certain chemicals, they light up, creating an electrical signal that the chip can process or amplify. Till now genetically engineered bacterium *Pseudomonas fluorescens* HK44 is used to create a biochip that is exquisitely sensitive to naphthalene, a common petroleum pollutant.

Table. 3: Biosensors used in pesticide detection based on the inhibition of enzymatic activity

Sl. No	Biological component	Transducer	Analyte
1	Acetylcholinesterase immobilized on multiwalled carbon nanotubes	Amperometry	Carbaryl
2	Acetylcholinesterase-choline oxidase on a gold-platinum bimetallic nanoparticles	Electrochemical impedance spectroscopy	Paraoxon ethyl, aldicarb and sarin
3	Acetylcholinesterase immobilized on polyaniline and multiwalled carbon nanotubes	Chronoamperometry	Carbaryl and methomyl

Table 4. Enzyme and detection method for heavy metal detection using biosensor

Sl. No.	Enzyme	Detection principle	Heavy metal
1	Acetylcholinesterase	Amperometry	Mercury
2	Alkaline phosphatase	Conductometry	Cadmium, cobalt, nickel and zinc
		Amperometry	Mercury, cadmium, zinc and copper
3	Glucose oxidase	Amperometry	Chromium

Biosensor for Identification of Contaminants in Water and Food

Food industry needs suitable analytical methods for process and quality control. Apart from identification of important analytes like sugars, alcohols, amino acids, flavours and sweeteners, it is very critical to identify the contaminants. The toxin namely ricin, botulinum toxins, saxitoxin, staphylococcal enterotoxin B, and trichothecene mycotoxins, are capable of being weaponized, and therefore early warning of possible exposure to these toxins is of great importance. *Bacillus cereus, Bacillus anthracis, Campylobacter jejuni*, cholera toxin, *Escherichia coli, Listeria monocytogenes, Salmonella typhimurium, Shigella* spp., *Staphylococcus aureus*, and *Staphylococcal enteritis* are just a few of the many types of pathogenic bacteria which are capable of infecting and harming humans.

The most common type of recognition element for these biosensors are antibodies/lectins, nucleic acid probes, aptamers, whole cells, and bacteriophages. Ricin can be identified using fluorescence array and SPR transducer using antibodies or oligosaccharides as recognizing element. Botulinum toxins have been detected mainly using the sandwich assay format utilizing antibodies with fluorescent tracers, antimicrobial peptides and aptamers. Staphylococcal enterotoxin B can be detected using antibody sandwich assay, SPR and piezoelectric crystal sensor. Cholera toxin is produced by the bacterium *Vibrio cholera* has been detected using antibodies/lectins in fluorescence, electrochemical and piezoelectric biosensor. *E. coli* has been detected using antibodies, antimicrobial peptides, aptamers, bacteriophages, β-galactosidase detection, and DNA probes using optical, electrochemical, and mass sensitive biosensors.

Pathogenic *Salmonella* has been detected using antibodies, antimicrobial peptides, bacteriophages, and DNA probes coupled with optical, electrochemical, and mass sensitive transduction techniques. *Staphylococcus aureus* was detected using antibodies and phages, and optical and mass sensitive techniques. Neurotoxic compounds like organophosphorus and non-organophosphorus can be detected using acetylcholinesterase and other cholinesterase enzymes as the biorecognition element through inhibition assays based on potentiometric, amperometric and piezoelectric transducers. The antinutritional compounds like oxalate, glycol-alkaloids or allergen (gluten) can be identified through amperometric and immunosensor, respectively.

Biosensor for Early Detection of Plant Diseases

The ability to detect, identify and quantify plant pathogens is very critical in plant pathology and nowadays biosensors are used to identify disease causing pathogens. Optical biosensor based on green fluorescent protein has been used for several plant pathogenic fungi detection like *Phytophthora palmivora, Ustilago maydis, Colletotrichum lindemuthianum, Aspergillus nidulans and Cochliobolus heterostrophus.* Chemiluminescent DNA optical fibre sensor for *Brettanomyces bruxellensis* detection was developed which produced neither false positives nor false negatives, and was both repeatable and faster with respect to traditional methods. A high sensitive menadione-catalyzed luminol chemiluminescent assay was developed for detection of fungi like *Saccharomyces cerevisiae, Candida maltose, Yarrowia lipolytica* and *Hansenula anomala.* Immunoassays like immunochromatographic strips and lateral flow devices make up most of the commercialized portable devices for plant disease diagnosis like *Spongospora subterranean* f. sp. *subterranean* causing powdery scab on potato tuber, *Pythium, Phytophthora, and Rhizoctonia.* Microfluidic immunosensor with micro-magnetic beads coupled to carbon-based screen-printed electrodes was used to detect *Botrytis cinerea.*

Conclusion

Overall, the use of biosensor in agriculture can provide a route to a specific, sensitive, rapid and inexpensive method of monitoring a range of analyte of interest. One of the important thing to be considered during designing and development of biosensor is that it can also be operated by a non-specialist person. With the development of technology there is still room for improvement of existing biosensors for real time detection and improved efficiency. Development of single biosensor with two or more transducing principles or one or two biorecognizing element for same analyte of interest will provide more qualitative dataset than conventional biosensor. With the advancements in nanobiotechnology, developments of new biological recognition element or synthetic material as recognition element can improve the detection limits of current biosensors used in agriculture. The next important thing is miniaturization using advanced fabrication procedures which can results in development of robust and inexpensive sensors. The demand for reliable and inexpensive methods for assessment is set to expand, and biosensors offer the opportunity to fulfill this niche.

Further Readings

Bhalla, N., Jolly, P., Formisano, N. and Estrela, P. 2016. Introduction to biosensors. Essays in Biochemistry, 60:1-8.

Terry, L.A. 2008. Agriculture, horticulture, and related applications. Part Eight. Biosensor Applications. In: Handbook of Biosensors and Biochips. Edited by R.S. Marks, D.C. Cullen, I. Karube, C.R. Lowe and H.H. Weetall. John Wiley & Sons, Inc., Eight:79.

Tothill, I.E. 2001. Biosensors developments and potential applications in the agricultural diagnosis sector. Computers and Electronics in Agriculture 30:205-218.

Velasco-Garcia, M.N. and Mottram, T. 2003. Biosensor technology addressing agricultural problems. Biosystems Engineering 84: 1-12.

Self-assessment Questions

1. Which of the following is a device to detect an analyte that combines a biological component with a physiochemical detector component?
2. (A) Biosensor (B) Sensor (C) Recognizing element (D) Output device
3. Biosensor consists of
4. (A) Sensitive biological element (B) Transducer (C) Detector (D) all the above
5. Which is the most widely used commercial biosensor
6. (A) Lipid biosensor (B) Glucose biosensor (C) Protein biosensor (D) all the above
7. Electrochemical biosensor is based on
8. (A) Radio frequency (B) Heat (C) Mass (D) Enzymatic catalysis
9. The application of biosensor includes

10. (A) Detection of food toxin (B) Detection of photosynthesis (C) Detection of micronutrient content in soil (D) Detection of soil organic carbon
11. Based on transducing principle, detection of analyte by change in their mass is called as........
12. Who is referred as Father of biosensor
13. .... feature of biosensor is called as the ability to generate identical responses for a duplicated experimental set-up.
14. Non-catalytic biosensor is classified into two types namely .... and ....
15. What does the abbreviation ELISA stand for? ....

Short answers

1. Define what the limit of detection is.
2. Explain how nitrogenous compound in soil and water are detected by biosensor technology.
3. Provide two examples of the use of enzymes as labels in biosensors.
4. Report an example of how whole cells could be used for biosensing.
5. Classify biosensor based on its activity

Brief answers

1. Describe the function of the biorecognition elements in a biosensor; list three different
2. biorecognition elements and describe how they can be used in biosensing.
3. How biosensor can be used in food industry
4. Describe and illustrate the working principle of a Quartz Crystal Micro balance (QCM) and explain one possible application in biosensing.
5. Explain the potential application of biosensor in identification of contaminants in soil and water
6. Explain the principle and various classifications of biosensor.

14

Nanotechnology Applications in Agriculture

Dr K S Subramanian, Dr K Raja & Dr C.R.Chinnamuthu,

Nanotechnology is a fascinating field of science dealing with a manipulation of atom by atom and thus products and processes evolved from nano science are the most précised ones that are impossible to achieve by the conventional systems. Nano particles are very tiny measuring a dimension of one-billionth of a metre (10^{-9} m) with extensive surface area. Despite nanotechnology being exploited in the fields of electronics, energy and health sectors, agricultural science is yet to make headway in achievements. It is an emerging field of science capable of resolving issues and problems that are unresolved in engineering and biological sciences. Among the advancement in science, nanotechnology is being visualized as a rapidly evolving field that has potential to revolutionize agriculture and food systems and improve the condition of the poor.

The Indian government is looking towards nanotechnology as a means of boosting agricultural productivity in the country. The Planning Commission of India recommended nanotechnology research and development (R&D) is one of six areas for investment. The commission recommended policies and carries out financial planning for government departments. The report was written by a subgroup of the commission, and incorporated into India's eleventh five-year plan, for 2007–2012. In order to harness the benefits of nanotechnology, biotechnology and bioinformatics to transform Indian agriculture, an exclusive National Institute of Nanotechnology in Agriculture has to be established. The report says nanotechnology such as nano-sensors and nano-based smart delivery systems could help ensure natural resources such as water, nutrients and chemicals are used efficiently in agriculture. Nano-barcodes and nano-processing could also help monitor the quality of agricultural produce. The report proposes a national consortium on nanotechnology R&D, to include the proposed national institute and Indian institutions that are already actively researching nanotechnology. It also recommended that Indian universities and institutions develop suitable graduate and postgraduate programs to train young scientists in nanotechnology. The International Food Policy Research Institute (IFPRI, 2011), Washington, suggested that inclusion of nanotechnology may improve crop productivity, reduces post-harvest losses, improves product quality, increasing the competitiveness of agricultural producers and improving market access. The advancement of nanotechnology may present new opportunities to improve the rural livelihoods of the poor.

Global Scenario

Nanotechnology is often referred as ***"Small Guys Big Business"***. The global nanotechnology market has touched US $29 billion mark in the year 2010 (Rs. 1,35,000 Crores) and it is currently US $ 2000 billion USD in 2017 (Rs. 13,40,000 crores). The investments are made in the order of materials (31%), electronics (28%), pharmaceuticals (17%), chemical manufacturing (9%), Aerospace (6%) and others (9%). Recent statistics suggests that 90% of the patents generated from just 7 countries comprising US, China, Germany, France, South Korea, Switzerland and Japan. The investment on agricultural sciences is well below 1% and therefore huge scope for agricultural scientists and industries to explore in the emerging field.

Indian Scenario

India's investment is far from the global club of nanotechnology. Various Ministries/Departments of Government of India such as the Department of Science and Technology (DST), Defense Research and Development Organization (DRDO), Council of Scientific and Industrial Research (CSIR) and Department of Biotechnology (DBT) have been supporting R&D in Nano Science and Technology. The DST launched the Nano Science and Technology Initiative (NSTI) in 2001 under the leadership of Prof. C. N. R. Rao. The NSTI has been focusing on research and development in nanoscience and technology in a comprehensive manner so that India can become a significant player in the area and contribute to the development of new technologies besides carrying out basic research at the frontiers of knowledge. The program supports R&D projects, strengthening of characterization and infrastructural facilities, creation of centres of excellence, generation of trained manpower, joint projects between educational institutions and industry for application development etc. The Government is embarking on plans for launching a Nano Science and Technology Mission (Nano Mission) has invested Rs. 1000 crore during 11th Five Year Plan (2007-2012) and it had nearly doubled during the 12th Five Year Plan (2013-2017) to further intensify its promotional efforts in this area. As part of the Nano Mission it is planned to launch a variety of educational and HRD programs, R&D programs, establish centers of excellence, promote institution-industry linked projects through increased public private partnerships, promoting entrepreneurship through establishment of business incubators, etc. The Nano Mission also plans to make special efforts for development and commercialization of nanotechnology, not only through public private partnerships but also by encouraging and enabling the private sector to invest in, and leverage, this sunrise technology.

Tamil Nadu Agricultural University

In India, the Tamil Nadu Agricultural University, Coimbatore, is one of the first State Agricultural Universities has initiated efforts to undertake research in the field of nanoscience. The TNAU has taken painstaking efforts to set up an exclusive Nanotechnology Center to accomplish the mission of "Nano Agriculture". Indian farming faces challenges such as shrinking arable lands, labour and water, exodus of people from farming, declining organic matter low fertilizer response ratio, resistance to GMOs and experiencing the fatigue of green revolution. To address all the challenges ahead, we should think of an alternate technology such as "nanotechnology" to precisely detect and deliver the correct quantity of nutrients or other inputs required by crops in suitable proportion that promote productivity while ensuring environmental safety.

In India, TNAU is an early bird in adopting the nanotechnology in order to gain the advantage of advancement made in the emerging field of science. The Nanotechnology Center in TNAU was established in 2010 with an initial investment of Rs. 12.0 crores on the state-of-the-art infrastructure facility, sophisticated equipments and human resource building. Twelve scientists of TNAU got trained in Nanotechnology from USA, Canada and Taiwan. Indeed, such efforts yielded fruition in setting up of the excellent fully equipped laboratory to undertake research in agricultural sciences. The Center is currently working on nano-inputs (nano-fertilizers, nano-herbicides, nano-pesticides, customized seeds), biosensors (early detection of diseases, mycotoxins and anti-nutritional factor), food systems (nano-films and nano encapsulation of functional foods) besides nano-remediation of pollutants in soil and aquatic systems. Our institute is fostering multi-faceted research collaborations with national and international organizations. We intend to provide advanced education and research opportunities to young graduates for taking the inventions from the laboratory to the farming community

Why do we need Nanotechnology in Indian Agriculture?

Indian agriculture is facing a wide spectrum of challenges in crop production systems such as crop yield stagnation, declining organic matter, multi-nutrient deficiencies, climate change, shrinking arable land, restructed labour and water availability and resistance to GMOs.

- Despite the fact that our research efforts for the past fifty years have helped us to achieve self-sufficiency food grain output, Indian agriculture begins to feel fatigue of green revolution recently and yields of many crops started stagnating. In 1950's the food grain production was just 50.5 million tonnes which had increased to 273 mt in 2017 and the country has to produce 300 mt by the year 2020 and 350 by 2030. Such an alarming increase in production requires out-of-box technologies and "nanotechnology" is being visualized as one of the emerging technology of choice. With the ever growing population in India, some alternate strategy to be evolved to producr more food grain from less and less amount of land, water and other resources.

- Indian soils are being exhausted heavily as 30 million tonnes of nutrients removed while 20 million tonnes added to crops leaving a net deficit of 10 million tonnes every year.
- Fertilizer response ratio of crops has declined drastically. For instance, we require 3.5 kg NPK nutrients to produce for every tonne of grain output in 1970's but currently 13.4 kg nutrients is necessary to havest the same amount of grains.
- Imbalanced fertilization is known to cause yield reductions besides environmental hazard. The NPK fertilizer ratio of 4:2:1 is ideal for crop productivity while the current ratio in India is being maintained at 10: 2.7: 1. This is due to the heavy subsidy to N fertiliers particularly, urea which is sold in the market half of the cost of manufacturing. The excessive use of N fertilizer affects groundwater and also causes eutrophication in aquatic ecosystems.
- In order to achieve a target of 300 million tonnes of food grains and to feed the burgeoning population of 1.5 billion in the year 2025, the country will require 45 million tonnes of nutrients as against a current consumption level of 23 million tonnes.
- Long-term fertilizer experiments conducted across the country has unequivocally demonstrated that conjunctive use of organic and inorganic is essential to sustain soil health. But the availability of organic manures is becoming scarce as a result of urbanization and reduction in animal wealth.
- Climate change is yet another serious concern. Eratic rainfall, frequent occuurence of drought, melting polar ice cap, temperature rise (0.4 to 4.0°C in the past century that coincides with increase in CO_2 concentration from 280 ppm in 1900 to 390 ppm in 2009) and declinining biodiversity.
- Crops are often exposed to abiotic (drought, salinity, nutrient deficiencies, heavy metal toxicities, high temperature) and biotic (pests, diseases, nematodes) stresses. There is a need for early detection of these factors in order to prepare the plants to tolerate sustain farm productivity.
- Socio-economic issues such as exodus of people from farming, non-availability of labourers and escalating cost of cultivation add enormous pressure on agricultural scientists to evolve technologies that target multi-faceted problems of Indian agriculture.
- To address all the challenges ahead, we should think of an alternate technology such as "nanotechnology" to precisely detect and deliver the correct quantity of nutrients or other inputs required by crops in suitable proportion that promote productivity while ensuring environmental safety.

Nano-fertilizers for Balanced Crop Nutrition

Fertilizers play a pivotal role in agricultural production. It has been unequivocally demonstrated that fertilizer contributes to the tune of 35-40% of the productivity of any crops. Without the fertilizer input, it is hardly possible to sustain agricultural productivity of our country. Considering its importance, the Government of India is heavily subsiding the cost of fertilizers particularly urea to encourage farmers to use them to promote productivity of crops. This resulted in imbalanced fertilization and occurrence of nitrate pollution in ground waters. In the past few decades, use efficiencies of N, P and K fertilizers remained constant as 30-35%, 18-20% and 35-40%, respectively, leaving a major portion of added fertilizers stay in the soil or enter into aquatic system causing eutrophication. The extent of multi-nutrient deficiencies are alarmingly increasing year by year which is closely associated with a crop loss of nearly 25-30%. The extent of nutrient deficiencies in the country are of the order of 89, 80, 50, 41, 49 and 33% for N, P, K, S, Zn and B, respectively. Thus from all sources, the country will be required to arrange for the supply of about 40-45mt of nutrients by 2025 (Subramanian and Tarafdar 2009).

Nano-fertilizers are nutrient carriers of nano- dimensions ranging from 30-40 nm (10^{-9} m or one- billionth of a metre) and capable of holding bountiful of nutrient ions due to their high surface area and release it slowly and steadily that commensurate with crop demand. Nano-fertilizers and nano-composites can be used to control the release of nutrients from the fertilizer granules so as to improve the nutrient use efficiency while preventing the nutrient ions either get fixed or lost to the environment. Nano-fertilizers have high use efficiency and can be delivered in a timely manner to a rhizospheric target. There are slow-release and super sorbent nitrogenous and phosphatic fertilizers. Some new- generation fertilizers have applications to crop production on long-duration human missions to space exploration.

According to the report of Iranian Nanotechnology Initiative Council (2009), Iranian researchers have produced the first nano-organic iron-chelated fertilizer in the world. Nano fertilizers have unique features like ultra high absorption, increase of 20 % to 200 % in production, rise in photosynthesis by 3.5 times and a 70% expansion in the leaves' surface area, Iranian Nanotechnology Initiative Council reported." While foreign samples cause an increase of up to 30 % in photosynthesis, the Iranian nano fertilizers are able to cause a 350% increase. Moreover, these nano fertilizers are environmentally sustainable due to their organic base, which makes them more suitable than foreign fertilizers that are hormone based.

The Tamil Nadu Agricultural University is one of the pioneering institutes initiated research in nano-fertilizers and the preliminary data are quite encouraging. Accordingly, zeolite based nano-fertilizers are capable of releasing nutrients especially NO_3-N more than 50 days while nutrient release from conventional fertilizer (urea) ceased to exist beyond 10-12 days (Subramanian et al., 2015). This suggests that nano-fertilizers may be used as a strategy to regulate the smart release of nutrients that commensurate with crop requirement. Research is underway to develop nano-composite to supply all the required essential nutrients in suitable proportion through smart delivery system. The impact of nano-fertilizer products on physiological, biochemical, nutritional and morphological changes in plants and the fate of nano-products in soil and plant systems have to be studied. In addition, the effects of nano-fertilizer products on rhizosphere microorganisms and biogeocycling of nutrients have to be explored.

Nitrogen

About 90% of Indian soils are deficient in N and thus there is a universal response for the addition of nitrogenous fertilizers. Indiscriminate use of N fertilizers caused major detrimental impacts on the diversity and functioning of the non-agricultural ecosystems due to eutrophication of freshwater and marine water. In addition, there can be gaseous emission of N reacting with the stratospheric ozone and the emission of toxic ammonia into the atmosphere. The nitrogen use efficiency (NUE) by crops is very low (30- 35%) due to the loss of N to the tune of 50 - 70% by leaching, volatalisation and microbial mineralization. One of the attempts to increase NUE is slow release or controlled release fertilizers which releases N slowly in available form or to develop materials which control the release of N in available form slowly. The most important slow release fertilizer is the coating of conventional N fertilizer with sulphur, neem, lac or clay. The idea was due to coating with these materials, urea comes into the soil solutions through diffusion process very slowly and in this way they supply nitrogen to the plants at a controlled rate or slow rate but for a longer period. But these attempts to increase the NUE were yielded with little success due to the mismatch between the nutrient release and crop demand. Nano-fertilizer may regulate the release of nutrients and deliver the correct quantity of nutrients required by the crops in suitable proportion and promote productivity while ensuring environmental safety.

Ammonium ions occupying the internal channels of zeolite is slowly set free, allowing the progressive absorption by the crop which results in a higher drymatter production of the crop. Zeolite impregnated with urea can be used as slow release fertilizer carrying the slow and steady release of N from nano-zeolite. Amending sandy soil with ammonium-loaded zeolite can reduce N leaching while sustaining growth of sweet corn and increasing N-use efficiency compared to ammonium sulphate.

In TNAU, Subramanian and Rahale (2009) have monitored the nutrient release pattern of nano-fertiliser formulations carrying nitrogen. The data have shown the nano-clay based fertilizer formulations (zeolite and montmorillonite with a dimension of 30-40 nm) are capable of releasing the nutrients for a longer period of time (>1000 hrs) than conventional fertilizers (< 500 hrs). Further, clay particles are adsorptive sites carrying reservoir of nutrient ions. Major portion of nutrient fixation occurs in the broken edges of the clay particles. Zero valence nano-particles can adsorb on to the clay lattice thereby preventing fixation of nutrient ions. Further, nano- particles prevent the freely mobile nutrient ions to get precipitated. These two processes assist in promoting the labile pool of nutrients that can be readily utilized by plants. Fertilizer particles can be coated with nano- membranes that facilitate in slow and steady release of nutrients. This process helps to reduce loss of nutrients while improving fertilizer use efficiency of crops.

The studies in the country and abroad have clearly shown that nanotechnology is shown to be promising in increasing the N use efficiency from 30-35% to 70% under laboratory conditions and the percentage increase may be little lower in open field conditions. Still it is a huge economic benefit to the country in terms of saving importing cost of fertilizers.

Nano-fertilizer with high N Use Efficiency

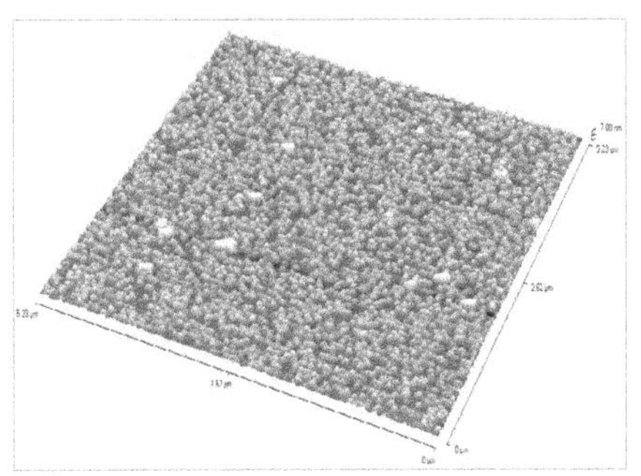

AFM picture showing Nano fertilizer

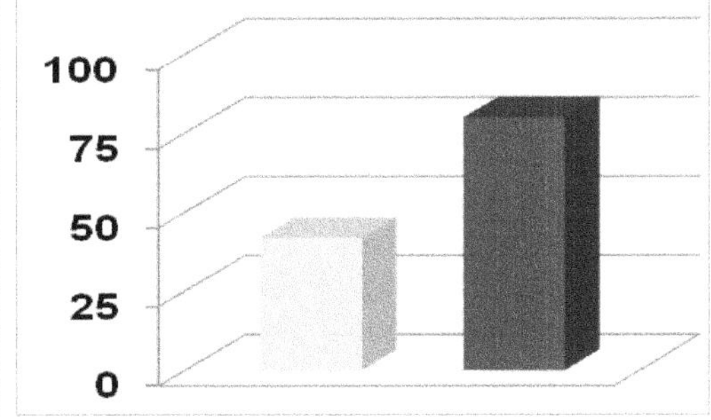

Relative performance of Nano-fertilizer

Phosphorus

Phosphorus (P) is a vital nutrient for plants because of its role in ribonucleic acid and function in energy transfers via ATP. It is often the limiting nutrient in agricultural ecosystems due to its low availability in soils. Phosphate ions in soil gets often fixed as Fe, Al and Ca in soils and a small fraction of phosphate in available form. The efficiency of fertilizer P use by crops ranged from 18 to 20 % in the year that it is applied. The remaining 78 to 80% becomes part of the soil P pool which is released to the crop over the following months and years. Polymer coating of mono ammonium phosphate (MAP) improved the plant recovery of fertilizer phosphorus (P) and provided a modest barley grain yield advantage relative to uncoated MAP. Coating P fertilizer could limit the contact of applied P with soil, possibly reducing its precipitation and/or adsorption on soil colloids, and increase its availability to developing plant roots. The development of thin polymer coatings has improved the opportunity to coat fertilizer granules and increased the predictability of when nutrients become available from the controlled-release product.

Recently, nano-zeolites are being used to regulate the nutrient release from the conventional phosphatic fertilizers. Since both zeolites and phosphate ions are negatively charged, zeolites surface has to be modified as the positively charged one using suitable surfactants. This process facilitates phosphates to adsorb on the surface modified zeolites to release slowly for an extended period of time. The release of P from fertilizer-loaded unmodified zeolite and surface modified zeolite (SMZ) and from solid KH_2PO_4 was performed using the constant flow percolation reactor. The results showed that the P supply from fertilizer-loaded SMZ was available even after 1080 h of continuous percolation, whereas P from KH_2PO_4 was exhausted within 264 h. The results indicated that SMZ is a good sorbent for

PO_4 and a slow release of suggested that SMZ has a great potential as the fertilizer carrier for slow release of P. In another study, mixing of rock phosphate (apatite) with zeolite is known to improve the availability of nutrients. The approximate reaction in soil solution is as follows:

$$(\text{P-rock}) + (NH_4 - \text{zeolite}) = (\text{Ca zeolite}) + (NH_4) + (H_2PO_4^-)$$

The zeolite takes Ca^{2+} from the phosphate rock, thereby releasing both phosphate and ammonium ions. Unlike the leaching of very soluble phosphate establish equilibrium. the fertilizers (for example, super phosphate), the controlled-release phosphate is released of a specific chemical reaction in soil. As phosphate is taken up by plants or by soil fixation, the chemical reaction releases more phosphate and ammonium in the attempt to reestablish equilibrium. The rate of phosphate release is controlled by varying the ratio of P-rock to zeolite. Phosphorus is also released from the rock by the lowering of soil pH as ammonium ions are converted to nitrate. Thus, the use of nano-zeolites can be potential factor in increasing the availability of both N and P simultaneously in soil solution in a regulated pattern.

Potassium

The common potassium fertilizers are completely water-soluble and, in some cases, have a high salt index. Consequently, when placed too close to seed or transplants, they can decrease seed germination and plant survival. This fertilizer injury is most severe on sandy soils, under dry conditions, and with high rates of fertilization – especially nitrogen and potassium. Some crops such as soybeans, cotton, and peanuts are much more sensitive to fertilizer injury than corn. There is little information available about potassium (K) use efficiency. However, it is generally considered to have a higher use efficiency than N and P because it is immobile in most soils and is not subject to the gaseous losses that N is or the fixation reactions that affect P. First year recovery of applied K can range from 20% to 60%. Improvement of nutrient efficiency in crops is an important issue in agriculture for reducing cost in agriculture production and for protecting the environment. Efficient use of nutrients is the relative ability of plant to produce maximal amounts of dry matter for each increment of nutrients accumulated or it is plant yield (productivity) per unit nutrient supply.

The high CEC of the nano-clays is caused by isomorphous substitution of silica (Si_4^+) with aluminum (Al_3^+) that eventually resulted in negative charge of the mineral lattice which attracts positive cationic nutrients. This negative charge is balanced by cations such as ammonium, sodium, calcium, and potassium, which are exchangeable with other cations. Such ion exchange assists in slow and steady release of K from nano-zeolite. Zeolites can become an excellent plant growth medium for supplying plant roots with additional vital nutrient cations and anions. The nutrients are provided in a slow-release, plant root demand-driven fashion through the process of dissolution and ion exchange reactions. The adsorption of nutrients by plant roots drives the dissolution and ion exchange reactions, pulling away nutrients as needed. The zeolite is then "recharged" by the addition of more dissolved nutrients. Their selectivity of ion exchange on zeolite was determined in an order of $K^+ > NH_4^+ > Na^+ > Ca_2^+ > Mg_2^+$.

Micronutrients

Micronutrients are elements which are essential for plant growth, but are required in much smaller amounts that include Fe, Mn, Cu, Zn, B and Mo. Micronutrient use efficiencies are very low in the range of 2-5% and rested of the added nutrients applied through fertilizers stay in the soil causing pollution. Natural zeolites, particularly clintopillolite have a high potential for Zn and Fe sorption with a high capacity for slow release fertilizers. Slow release of Zn is attributed to the sparingly solubility of minerals and sequestration effect of exchanger, there by releasing trace nutrients to zeolite exchange sites where they are more readily available for uptake by plants. The release of cationic micronutrients has enhanced in the presence of zeolite in neutral soil. There were attempts to convert conventional micronutrient fertilizers into nano-forms using top down approaches wherein size of the particles were reduced by high energy ball milling for 4-6 hrs at 600 rpm. Zinc oxide nano- particles were shown to improve the growth of the plants as nano-ZnO can enter the root tissue of rye grass directly and improve the germination. Such translocation of nano-particles in in plant system has been visualized using high resolution imaging using TEM and fluorescence microscopy. In another approach, Zn ions have been encapsulated into manganese core shell to minimize the precipitation of Zn. This process has increased the Zn use efficiency from 3% to 6% and enhanced the productivity of rice under greenhouse conditions.

Nanocomposites

Nano-composites have been developed in order to supply wide range of nutrients in desirable properties. These compounds are capable of regulating the inputs depending on the conditions of soil or requirement of crops. Zinc–aluminium layered double- hydroxide nano-composites have been used for the controlled release of nutrients that regulate plant growth. In soil niches, nano-materials are porous and hydrated and as such they control moisture retention, permeability, solute transport, and availability of plant nutrients in soils. These nano-materials materials also control exchange reactions of dissolved inorganic and organic species between the soil solution and colloidal surfaces. The physico-chemical properties in the surface of nano-composites provide much of reactivity to soil biological and abiotic processes. Organic material intercalation with natural kaoline exfoliated into nanometer sized layers serve as a composite to retain and release a wide array of nutrients. The organic agent and clays formed nano-composites through hydrogen bond combination. The SEM pictures of polystyrene-starch nano-subnano composites showed that many pores were present on the surface of film at sizes ranging from 10 to 20 nm. These nano- subnano composites were used as the cementing and coating materials of slow/controlled release fertilizer.

Nano-fertilizers on soil health and crop productivity

Nano-fertilizers have been tested in rice, maize and groundnut. In all the cases, nutrient use efficiencies had been increased from 25-50% which is considered as the saving of fertilizer input. Further, nano-fertilizer has increased the yield by 10-40% without associated ill-effects. Nano-fertilizer applied soil had higher available status of nutrients than conventional fertilizer applied soil. In rice, encapsulated Zn could increase the yield by 30% even under constraints of moisture with an added advantage of biofortification of Zn in grains. In maize, N use efficiency had doubled when urea is intercalated with nano-zeolite. Nano-S fertilizer has higher use efficiency by 10% than gypsum fertilized groundnut plants. Further, nano-S fertilized plants had higher concentrations of S in the nodules, kernels and leaves. The data suggest that nano-S can facilitate targeted delivery of S in plant systems but mechanisms involved are poorly understood.

Cross Section of Root Nodules Fertilized with Nano-S

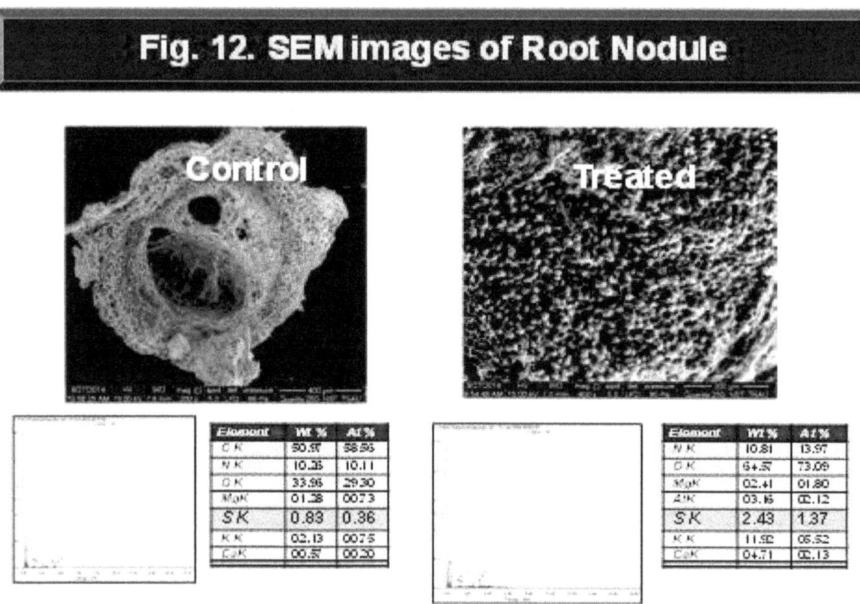

Root Nodules of Nano-S fertilized Groundnut Plants

2. Nano-particles for Seed Invigouration

Seed is a basic input deciding the fate of productivity of any crop. Conventionally, seeds are analyzed for their germination and distributed to farmers for sowing. Despite the fact that the germination percentage registered in the seed testing laboratory is about 80-90%, it hardly happens in the field due to the inadequacy or non-availability of sufficient moisture under rainfed system. In India, more than 70% of the net area sown is under rainfed system, it is quite appropriate to develop technologies for rainfed agriculture. Seed coating or hardening techniques have been optimized and extensively studied for a wide array of crops and evolved strategies to ensure germination. This process will make the seed hardened and emerge faster besides withstanding early drought. Though it is a useful strategy but rarely adopted by farmers due to practical difficulties. This necessitates evolving an alternate and innovative method to tackle the issue of poor germination in rainfed system. Recently, some preliminary works have been done in order to improve the emergence of seed utilizing a wide array of nano-particles and metal oxides.

Carbon nano-tubes (CNTs) are nanomaterials widely used in biological and material sciences. Single and multi-walled carbon nano-tubes are commercially available to carryout smart delivery of water, nutrients and medicines etc. Since CNT carries extensive surface area, they have the potential to regulate the moisture under constraints of irrigation or drought conditions. Khodakovskaya and her team in 2009 at the University of Arkansas, USA, have used carbon nano-tube for improving the germination of tomato seeds. In this elegant experimental system, the substrate impregnated with differential quantities of carbon nano-tubes. The data have vividly shown that there is a direct relationship between the quantities of CNT and rate of germination. The authors suggest that CNT serves as new pores for water permeation by penetration of seed coat. Further, the CNT can act as a gate to channelize the water from the substrate in to the seeds. The situation can be mimicked in rainfed system wherein moisture is constraint can be tide over through the CNTs. Indeed, CNTs had shown to improve the germination and seedling vigour of several crop species such as wheat, oat, barley, soybean, tomato, onion and lucerne.

The metal oxide NPs like ZnO is known to improve the germination and seedling vigor of a wide spectrum of crops such as tomato, onion, chilli, groundnut and blackgram. In all the cases, the improved germination is resulted from the quenching of reactive oxygen species that are emanated during storage. On entry of the ZnO into the seeds, the ZnO undergoes dissociation which eventually resulted in quenching reactive oxygen species that closely coincided with cell membrane integrity. Further, Zn as a nutrient it can assist in promoting growth hormones in the germinating. In *Cicer arietinum*, Pandey *et al.* (2010) found that ZnO NPs increased the level of IAA in the roots (sprouts) and thereby an increase in the growth rate of plants was observed. Consequently, ZnO NPs has improved the germination, seedling growth and vigour index in blackgram. Pulses seeds dressed with ZnO NPs @ 1000 mg kg^{-1} found to increase the germination under *in vitro* conditions.

Silver (Ag) nano-particles are widely used in agri-food systems. These NPs are well known for their anti-microbial properties. As a result of anti-microbial and anti-pathogenic effects, seed borne pathogens are effectively controlled that eventually has resulted in improved germination of many crop species such as maize, beans, cowpea, watermelon and zucchini. Despite the fact that Ag NPs are beneficial, excessive use is reported to have deleterious effects on crops. Ag NPs showed a toxic effect on corn root elongation. This study showed that exposure to Ag NPs caused both positive and negative effects on plant growth and germination.

In addition to ZnO, TiO_2 NPs are found to have favourable effects on seed invigoration. On entry to the seeds, TiO_2 NPs quench the reactive oxygen species and break the dormancy caused by the phenolics in the seeds. TiO_2 NPs treatment @ 60 ppm improved the germination in *Foeniculum vulgare*. TiO_2 NPs enhanced the seed germination and promoted radicle and plumule growth of canola seedlings. Zero valent Iron (ZVI) NPs also exhibited similar effects in several crops.

Other NPs such as copper, silica, alumina and cerium had reported to improve germination of a wide array of crops. In most cases, the entry of NPs led to the donation of electron and pairing of unpaired electrons which ultimately caused the repair of damage caused by lipid peroxidation. In addition, these NPs have anti-microbial properties which facilitate protection against seed borne pathogens.

Overall, the NPs have potential beneficial effects in enhancing the seed quality by circumventing oxidative damages caused by seed deterioration. The mechanisms underlying on NPs induced enhancement of seed germination. Optimal use of NPs can help to improve the germination and seedling vigour without associated ill-effects. On the other hand, excessive use has deleterious impacts especially for ZnO and Ag NPs. Care should be taken to gain the benefits of nano-particles while impeding the ill-effects of excess use. More research is required to commercialize NPs use in seed invigoration.

Several decades of seed research provided insights into the mechanisms relating to the seed quality that closely coincided with the development of invigouration techniques. Indeed, none other than seed as an input has a direct relevance in sustaining the farm productivity and profitability. In India, traditionally, seeds of the previous season will serve as an input for succeeding cropping season. Currently, there is a paradigm shift from the use of owned seed source to procurement from the market. The span between the cropping decision and procurement of seeds from authentic source is very narrow and hardly possible for the Indian farmers to check the seed quality prior to sowing. This situation necessitates infusing innovative technologies and techniques for quick detection of seed quality and invigoration of seed lots using customized materials. These innovative technologies are often referred as the third generation seed treatments for quality enhancement and assurance that encompass seed quality detection using e-nose, nano-barcoding, high resolution imaging, seed quality enhancement using customized nano-particles, seed coating and smart delivery of agri-inputs through seeds. Since, seed is a "nano-input" and a miniaturized laboratory that can serve as a single solution to address complex and multi-dimensional field problems.

Application of Nanotechnology for Rainfed Agriculture

More than 60% of agriculture is rainfall dependent and soil moisture decides the fate of productivity of crops. Several drought management strategies such as mulching, organic manuring, soil hybridization, use of super absorbents, anti-transpirants besides inclusion of tolerant varieties are being recommended. These practices have been tested over the past several decades but found futile as the intensity and occurrence of drought varies with location and the coincidence of critical stage of crop water requirement. This situation warrants infusion of innovative technologies such as nanotechnology wherein the design and fabrication of moisture conservation inputs is possible by atom-by-atom manipulation and demand-driven smart delivery.

Soil breeding is well known practice wherein heavy textured clay soil is blended in light (sandy) soils in order to improve the physical fertility thereby moisture conservation is achieved. Despite the practice is very effective, farmers could not afford to adopt due to heavy investments on transport of bulky materials. With a view to reduce the bulkiness while taking advantage of clays, nano-clays have been widely studied as a measure to mitigate drought. Application of nano clay improved the water holding capacity of sandy soils in Egypt. Further, intercalation of Zn coated nano-clays with polyacrylamide polymer can improve moisture conservation in rain fed rice. Nano-clay polymer Composite (NCPC) increased the water holding capacity besides served as a slow release formulation for nutrients. Recently, scientists have attempted to spray the montmorillionite nanoclays on the soil that facilitates aggregate stability which eventually resulted in improving the moisture retention capacity of the soil.

Òrganic polymers possess unique property of holding moisture several times as that of their weight. One such acrylamide based super absorbent polymers was introduced in late 1980's and tested in rainfed agriculture. A super-absorbent polymer (Jalshakthi) introduced in 1990's was found to increase the gravimetric moisture content in sandy loam soil (Alfisol) but the moisture release to the rainfed sunflower was hardly achieved due to the retention of soil moisture at high atmospheric pressure. Recently, nanotechnology approaches are being employed to enhance the moisture retention and regulated release which coincides with crop water demand. Further, hydrophobic nano-polymeric materials can be used as a cover to conserve moisture while preventing drainage loss. Superabsorbent polymers with a complex of carboxy methly cellulose and starch cross-linked with aluminum are reported to retain 73% higher moisture. In addition to organic polymers, inorganic complex such as Iron oxalate capped iron-oxide (OCIO) nano-materials can improve water retention in soils by reducing bulk density and improving soil aggregation. Blending of organic (polyacrylic acid and carboxy methyl cellulose) and inorganic (montmorillonite) compounds to develop nano-composites to enhance moisture retention and release characteristics of soil.

3. Nano-herbicides

Weeds are menace in agricultural production system. Since two-third of Indian agriculture is rainfed farming where usage of herbicide is very limited, weeds have the potential to jeopardize the total harvest in the delicate agro-ecosystems. Non-availability of labours in rainfed areas is a serious cause for concern. Among the weed species, nut grass (*Cyperus rotundus*) is one of the most notorious weeds very difficult to eradicate due to the fact that this weed species produces tuber that carries large amounts of starch. The herbicides available in the market mostly target above ground parts particularly the foliage. As a result, tuber in the underground rejuvenates and emerges out in the successive days and reduces the efficacy of herbicides.

Under rainfed conditions, there is no guarantee for moisture availability and thus herbicides are to be designed and fabricated to release the active ingredient only when the soil receives a short spell of rainfall. Nanotechnology can be employed to synthesize smart herbicides that release active herbicide molecules only when moisture is available in rainfed system besides targeting both leaves and tubers. The existing herbicide molecules can be encapsulated with a suitable hydrophilic polymers such as Poly styrene sulfonate (PSS) and poly allylamine hydrochloride (PAH)) that facilitate the release of herbicide molecules synchronize with soil moisture which circumvent weed seeds from germinating. Nano-herbicides are quite ideal for rainfed farming where weed menace is harder to overcome.

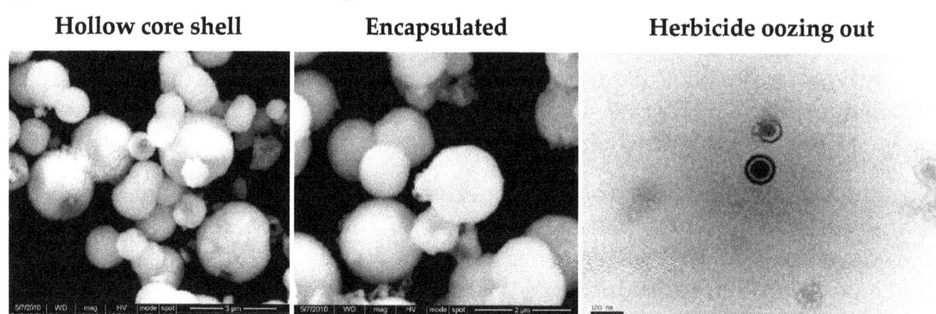

Sequential steps Involved in Encapsulation of Herbicides

Nano-capsulated herbicides are known to control the notorious parasitic weeds while reducing the phytotoxicity of herbicides on crops that explains the benefits of smart delivery system in agriculture. Properly functionalized nano-capsules provide better penetration through cuticle and allow slow and controlled release of active ingredients on reaching the target weed. Nano encapsulation of chemicals with biodegradable materials makes safer and easy to handle by the growers. Efforts are underway to kill the notorious weeds like *Cyprus rotundus* through smart delivery system. This weed produces tubers rich in starch that has to be exhausted through a suitable smart delivery system. Nano-encapsulated agrochemicals should be designed in such a way that they possess all necessary properties (effective concentration, stability and solubility) time controlled release in response to certain stimuli, enhanced targeted activity and less eco-toxicity with safe and easy mode of delivery thus avoiding repeated applications.

- **Nanotechnology to manage problem weeds**: Develop a receptor based herbicide molecule targeting to kill underground propagules. Several pesticide manufacturers are developing agrochemicals encapsulated in nanoparticles. If the active ingredient is combined with a smart delivery system, herbicide will be applied only when necessary according to the conditions present in the field. These chemicals may be time released or released upon the occurrence of an environmental trigger (for example, temperature, humidity and light).

- **Nano-herbicides to exhaust the weed seed bank:** Molecular characterization of problem weed seed coat will help us to identify the receptor having specific binding property with nanoherbicide molecules.
- **Nano-herbicides to eradicate the perennial weed** Nanotechnology has a potential for efficient delivery of chemicals using nano-sized preparations or nano-materials based agrochemical formulations.
- Nanotech approach will reduce the need for toxic herbicides, which many weed species have grown resilient to. By using nanoherbicide which is 1-100 nm range will try to mingle with the soil particle and try to destroy the entire weeds from their roots by not affecting other food crops.

Due to incredibly small proportions of nano-scale herbicides, then can easily blend with soil and attack seeds that are buried below the reach of tillers and conventional herbicides. As the nanoparticles are target specific they can be used to kill the weeds and destroy it to get better yield. Herbicides like atrazine, triazine could be encapsulated to get efficient release to the plants.

Detoxification of herbicide residue: Nanoscale iron particles have large surface areas and high surface reactivity. They provide enormous flexibility in *insitu* applications. Research has shown that nanoscale iron particles can be effectively used for the transformation and detoxification of a wide variety of common environmental contaminants such as chlorinated organic solvents and chlorinated pesticides. Modified iron nanoparticles, such as catalyzed nanoparticles have been synthesized further to enhance the speed and efficiency of remediation.

Atrazine has high persistence (half life-125 days in sandy soils) and mobility in some types of soils because it is not easily absorbed by soil particles and often causes contamination of soil and groundwater. Based on the preliminary study (under laboratory condition) at TNAU it was found that Silver modified Ferric Oxide (Fe_3O_4) - CMC nanoparticles was superior in degrading the atrazine. They showed 82-88 % degradation of atrazine. Further studies are required to standardize the synthesis of iron based metal nanoparticle and nanocomposite for higher surface reactivity, stabilizing with suitable capping agent for sustaining the reaction under different agro ecosystem.

Nanotechnology for Plant Protection

Persistence of insecticides in the initial stage of crop growth helps in bringing down the pest population below economic threshold level and to have an effective control for a longer period. Hence, the persistence of pesticides is one of the most cost-effective and versatile means of controlling insect pests. In order to protect the active ingredient from the environmental conditions and to promote persistence, a nanotechnology approach "encapsulation (nano / micro)" can be used to improve the insecticidal value. Microencapsulation comprises nano-sized particles of the active ingredients being sealed by a thin-walled sac or shell (protective coating).

In Tamil Nadu agricultural University, neem-based nano emulsion (~200 nm) has been developed and found effective in controlling sucking pests such as thrips, aphids and mites in Chillies. Recently, several research papers have been published on the encapsulation of insecticides. Nanoencapsulation of pesticides allows for proper absorption of the chemical into the plants unlike the case of conventional formulations. Nano-encapsuation of insecticides, fungicides or nematicides will help in producing nano-formulations which offer effective control of pests while preventing residues in soil.

In addition to the encapsulated forms of insecticides, some of the nano-particles are being used as effective strategy to protect the crops from the damage by pests and diseases. Surface modified hydrophobic nanosilica has been successfully used to control a range of agricultural pests. This functionalized lipophilic nanosilica gets absorbed into the circular lipids of insects by physiosorption and damages the protective wax layer and induces death by desiccation. The use of such nano-biopesticide is more acceptable since they are safer for plants and cause less environmental pollution in comparison to conventional chemical pesticides.

The successful use of silver nano-particles (Ag NPs) in diverse medical streams as antifungal and antibacterial agents has led to their applications in controlling phytopathogens. Ag NPs with broad spectrum of antimicrobial activity reduce various plant diseases caused by spore producing fungal pathogens. The effectiveness of Ag NPs can be improved by applying them well before the penetration and colonization of fungi within the plant tissues. The small size of the active ingredient effectively controls fungal diseases like powdery mildew. However, it was also observed that a very high concentration of nano-silica-silver produced chemical injuries on the cucumber. The use of Ag NPs as an alternative to fungicides for the control of sclerotium forming phytopathogenic fungi was also investigated. Exposure of fungal hyphae to Ag NPs caused severe damage by the separation of layers of hyphal wall and collapse of hyphae. The efficacy of Ag NPs in extending the vase life of gerbera flowers was also studied and the results show inhibited microbial growth and reduced vascular blockage which increased the water uptake and maintained the turgidity of gerbera flowers. Apparently, the use of biocide containing polymeric nanoparticles for introducing organic wood preservatives and fungicides into wood products thereby reducing the wood decay was also studied. Among the nano-particles, Ag NPs are widely used accounting for more than 30 per cent of the nano-based commercial products in the world. The use of nano-particles in plant protection and production is summarized in Table

Smart Delivery Systems in Agriculture

Nanoscale devices are envisioned that would have the capability to detect and treat diseases, nutrient deficiencies or any other maladies in crops long before symptoms were visually exhibited. "Smart Delivery Systems" for agriculture can possess timely controlled, spatially targeted, self-regulated, remotely regulated, pre-programmed, or multi-functional characteristics to avoid biological barriers to successful targeting. Smart delivery systems can monitor the effects of delivery of nutrients or bioactive molecules or any pesticide molecules. This is widely used in health sciences wherein nanaoparticles are exploited to deliver required quantities of medicine to the place of need in human system. In the smart delivery system, a small sealed package carries the drug which opens up only when the desirable location or infection site of the human or animal system is reached. This would allow judicious use of antibiotics than otherwise would be possible. A molecular-coded "address label" on the outside of the package could allow the package to be delivered to the correct site in the body. Similarly, implanting nano-particles in the plants could determine the nutrient status in plants and take up suitable remedial measures well before the malady causes yield reduction in crops. The fertilizer or irrigation requirement of crops can be scouted by nanotechnology. The exciting possibility of combining agricultural science and nanoscale technology into sensors holds the potential of increased sensitivity and therefore a significantly reduced response-time to sense field problems. "Smart" delivery systems could contain on-board chemical detection and decision making capability for self-regulation that could deliver active chemical molecules or nutrients as needed. Remote activation and monitoring of intelligent delivery systems can assist agricultural growers of the future to minimize antibiotic and pesticide use.

Role of Nanotechnology in Precision Farming

Precision farming has been a long-desired goal to maximize output (i.e. crop yields) while minimizing input (i.e. fertilizers, pesticides, herbicides etc.) through monitoring environmental variables and applying targeted action. Precision farming makes use of computers, global satellite positioning systems, and remote sensing devices to measure highly localized environmental conditions thus determining whether crops are growing at maximum efficiency or precisely identifying the nature and location of problems. By using centralized data to determine soil conditions and plant development, seeding, fertilizer, chemical and water use can be fine-tuned to lower production costs and potentially increase production – all benefiting the farmers. Precision farming can also help to reduce agricultural waste and thus keep environmental pollution to a minimum. Although not fully implemented yet, tiny sensors and monitoring systems enabled by nanotechnology will have a large impact on future precision farming methodologies.

One of the major roles for nanotechnology-enabled devices will be the increased use of autonomous sensors linked into a GPS system for real-time monitoring. These nanosensors could be distributed throughout the field where they can monitor soil conditions and crop growth. Nanosensors utilizing carbon nanotubes or nano-cantilevers are small enough to trap and measure individual proteins or even small molecules. Nanoparticles or nanosurfaces can be engineered to trigger an electrical or chemical signal in the presence of a contaminant such as bacteria. Other nanosensors work by triggering an enzymatic reaction or by using nanoengineered branching molecules called dendrimers as probes to bind to target chemicals and proteins. Ultimately, precision farming, with the help of smart sensors, will allow enhanced productivity in agriculture by providing accurate information, thus helping farmers to make better decisions.

The nanotechnology is an emerging field of science can be exploited to derive solution to a wide range of unsolved field problems. The Department of Nano Science & Technology, Tamil Nadu Agricultural University, Coimbatore, is currently working on nano-fertilizer, nano-herbicide, nano-pesticide, nano-seed science, nano-encapsulation of functional foods, nano-packaging to preserve fruits and vegetables, biosensor for early detection of plant diseases and nano-remediation of soil and aquatic pollutants.

Nanotechnology is a fascinating field of science widely exploited in various disciplines and this book chapter highlighted that how best the tools and techniques can be employed in agricultural sciences to promote productivity without associated impacts on environment. Nanoscience and technology is being visualized to revolutionize agriculture sector in the years to come. The futuristic agriculture should focus on the development of processes and products intended to deliver inputs precisely, besides deriving solution to unresolved issues at the farm gate. The use efficiency of agricultural inputs hardly exceeds 25-30% and major portion gets wasted and the research efforts taken to tide over the problems in the past few decades did not exhibit any fruitful results. This necessitates for an alternate strategy of infusing nanotechnology in agricultural sector to enhance input use efficiency within the complex environmental conditions. Despite nanotechnology applications in agriculture is just beginning to surface, the reported literature review has vividly indicated that there is a vast scope of inclusion of nanotechnology in developing smart delivery of agricultural inputs such as fertilizers, seed invigoration chemicals, pesticides, soil moisture conservation amendments besides developing diagnostic kits and tools for early detection of diseases, pests, moisture status and quality of crop produce. In order to augment the research efforts in nanotechnology, agricultural scientists should take a hue from medical sciences which serve as a guiding force that can be exploited in agricultural production systems. In this book chapter, the literature review made has clearly suggest that there is an abundance of scope to exploit smart delivery of agricultural inputs which facilitate enhanced use efficiency and ensure environmental protection.

Self-assessment Questions

1. Why do we need nano-fertilizer ?
2. Which is the most commonly used substrate for nano-fertilizer ?
3. Do Indian farmers benefit from nanotechnology ?
4. What is smart delivery of nutrients ?
5. How does CNTs improve germination ?
6. Role of ZnO in seed invigoration ?
7. What is encapsulated herbicide ?
8. Commonly used polymers for moisture dependent release of herbicide

9. What is hydrogel ?
10. Will the nano-products be cost-effective ?
11. Define co-acervation
12. Uniqueness of nano-pesticides
13. Do the nano-products safer to environment
14. What is precision farming?
15. Define "Rhizosphere".

15

Applications of Nanotechnology in Food Systems

Dr Haripriya Shanmugam

Diet-related health issues continue to increase globally based on the behavior of foods, as they are processed within the human digestive system. The food industry is focusing on developing beneficial functional foods as prophylactic measure for healthy-living. Nanotechnology is revolutionizing the entire food system from production to processing, storage and product development. Understanding the nature of food and food processing at the nanoscale level is important to create new and improved food products. Characteristics of food change at nano dimension *i.e.,* food texture, taste, colour, and stability during processing and storage. In addition, nanotechnology can also improve aqueous/water solubility, thermal stability and oral bioavailability of food active ingredients. At present, nanotechnology is applied towards developing nanocomposites in food packaging material (for controlling diffusion of food. Food active ingredients and protection from microbial attack), nanobiosensors (for detection of food contamination and quality deterioration) and nanoencapsulation of food active ingredients (for better delivery of nutraceuticals).

Natural Nanostructures in Food

Natural foods do contain nanoscale components within them and the functional properties of food are determined by their structure. Proteins in food are globular in structure ranged from 10 to several 100 nm, while polysaccharides and lipids are less than one nm in thickness. Milk and milk products naturally contain nanostructures like milk proteins (beta-lactoglobulin), casein micelles and whey protein. When our food is subject to cooking/processing, nanostructures are produced, e.g. coagulation, emulsification, homogenization and milling. When starch is boiled to make custard, three-dimensional crystalline structures (10nm in thickness) are formed. When milk is homogenized, fat globules of 100 nm sized droplets are produced. Naturally occurring nanostructures in food improve functional behavior of the food.

A suitable example is milk in liquid phase can be converted into multiphase structures like gels, emulsions, foams and powders depending on the processing methods. Structural complexities of foods lead to development of food products with different structures, functions and palatability.

Nanoencapsulation of Food Bioactives

An important application of nanotechnology in food and nutrition is to develop novel functional food ingredients with improved water solubility, oral bioavailability, acceptable sensory attributes and stability during food processing and storage. Currently, food active ingredients like minerals (Iron, calcium), carotenoids (β-carotene and lycopene), vitamins (Vitamin D, thiamin, riboflavin), essential fatty acids (omega 3) and antioxidants (polyphenolic compounds) are gaining significance towards developing functional foods/nutraceuticals. However, oral administration of food active ingredients in pure form often results in poor systemic bioavailability (amount of food active ingredient actually absorbed by the body) as well as instability in the gastrointestinal tract (pH and presence of enzymes). Poor aqueous solubility of food active ingredients limits the efficacy of the molecule inside the body. Likewise, instability of food active ingredients is also encountered during food processing and storage due to auto-oxidation, photo-oxidation and thermal degradation.

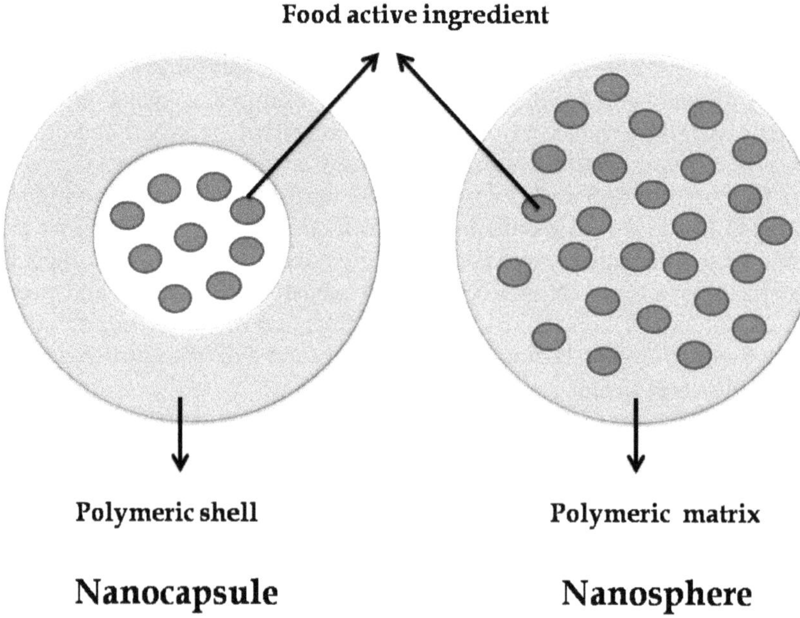

Fig. 1: Graphical representation of nanostructure formed with food active ingredient and polymeric wall material (Credit: Haripriya Shanmugam and Preetha Sundharam)

Nanoencapsulation is a technique used to improve oral bioavailability, provide protection from adverse environmental factors during storage and for controlled/

prolonged release of food active ingredients. Nanoencapsulation is a method of incorporation of food active ingredients in nanostructured vesicles or wall materials (Fig 1.). The wall material should be food-grade biopolymers like proteins, polysaccharides and lipids to produce nanostructures. Nanoencapsulation works well, because delivery of any food active ingredient within the body is directly affected by particle size. By reducing the particle size to nano regime, solubility of food active ingredients can be improved through an increase in surface area-to-volume ratio, thereby improved oral bioavailability. Food active ingredients that are nanoancapsulated to overcome bioavailability and stability issues are listed in Table 1. Besides improving bioavailability, nanoencapsulation also offers additional advantages like ease in handling, retention of flavor compounds, taste masking, triggered/controlled/prolonged release for long-lasting organoleptic perception.

Table 1. Nanoencapsulation of food actives ingredients suitable with wall material for desirable Functionality

Food bioactives	Wall material	Advantages
Curcumin	Casein complex micelle	Increased aqueous solubility and antioxidant activity
Resxevatrol	Gelatin complex	Increased aqueous solubility and stability
Epigallactocatechin gallate	β-Lactoglobulin complex	Decrease degradation due to hydrolyzing enzymes
β-carotene	Palmitic acid- Corn oil	Improved chemical stability
Quercetin	Glycerol monostearate	Improved bioavailability
Melatonin	Cholesterol, Phosphatidylcholine	Improved bioavailability
Rosemary oil	Gum arabic	Improved flavour retention upto 30%
Chlorogenic acid	Soy bean lecithin + Cholesterol	Reduced degradation and high anti-oxidant activity
Caffeic acid	β-cyclodextrin	High solubility and Photostability
Orange oil	Gum arabic	Improved oil retention
Vannillin	Poly vinyl alcohol + Cyclodextrin	Improved retention and stability

Nanosensors for Food Quality Assessment

Amount of glucose, fructose, sucrose, D-sorbitol, L-malic acid, citric acid, succinic acid, L-glutamic acid, hydrogen peroxide and alcohol formed during food processing and storage is used as an indicator of food quality. For artificial sensing, electronic nose (a device that identifies specific volatile components of an odor) and electronic tongue (array of sensors immersed in liquids to identify different physico-chemical characteristics relevant to tastes) are developed to increase the sensitivity of such chemical detection. With advancement in microelectromechanical systems (MEMS) and nanoelectromechanical systems (NEMS), different nanostructured materials are successfully used in fabrication of such sensing devices with increased sensitivity (in parts per trillion). High surface area to volume ratio of the nanomaterials is advantageous for sensor applications, as most of the sensing part has to interact with the target analytes present in food. Feasible application of nanomaterial based e-nose and e-tongue for food quality assessment are listed in Table 2.

Process of producing specialty edible produces hike cheese making, brewing and wine production has relied on human senses to assess its quality for a long period of time. For example, organoleptic property of wine (flavour) are determined by more than 800 volatile organic compounds arising from grapes and/or formed during fermentation process. The abundance of volatile organic compounds depends on grape variety and origin, processing practices comprising blending, aging and in particular, on the nature of yeast used for fermentation, postproduction treatment and storage, which ultimately decides the product quality. Functionally, antioxidant capacity of red wine depends on its phenolic content, which decides the beneficial health property. Tyrosinase enzyme immobilized gold nanoparticle modified glassy carbon electrode was used to detect the quality of phenol in red and white wines from grapes. Likewise, gold nanoparticles immobilised pyranose oxidase has been used for detection of glucose in fruit juices like orange, peach, pomegranate and mixed fruit. Gold nanoparticles ensure desirable catalytic activity and analytical performance of the biosensor. Fast response time, high sensor response and detection at very low concentrations are some of the advantages of nanosciences. However, development of e-tongue and e-nose based on nanomaterials is still a challenge.

Table 2. Application of e-tongue and e-nose with enhanced nano sensitivity for food quality Assessment

Type of sensing device	Applications in food Industry
Electronic nose	➢ Differentiate contaminated and uncontaminated milk
	➢ Detect mycotoxins present in wheat grains
	➢ Predict fruit maturity indices.
	➢ Identification of adulteration in virgin coconut oil
Electronic tongue	➢ Flavor ageing in beverages (fruit juice, alcoholic or non-alcoholic drinks and flavored milks)
	➢ Quantify bitterness or "spicy level" of drinks or dissolved compounds (Tea samples)
	➢ Control ageing process of cheese and whiskey

Detection of Food Microbial Contamination

Food quality assessment can be generally evaluated by monitoring the presence of pesticides, pathogens and mycotoxins, toxins, food contaminants depending on type of spoilage and adulterations. Food contaminated with microbes and adulteration can cause serious health problems and their detection in foods at low concentration is quite challenging. Integration of the nanomaterial in the biosensor assembly for faster electron transfer of enzymes as well as higher specificity for analyte (in food sample) has shown great promises in the food industry. Various forms of nanomaterials like gold and quantum dot nanoparticles, single and multiwalled carbon nanotubes immobilized with enzymes has been employed for the checking the quality of food samples. Presence of *Escherichia coli* in milk was detected using amine-functionalized magnetic nanoparticles. Aflatoxins are a group of toxic and carcinogenic compounds found in food contaminated with *Aspergillus flavus* and *Aspergillus parasiticus*. Gold nanoparticles immobilised with aflatoxin oxidase has been used as sensor for the detection of aflatoxin B1. Likewise, citrate-coated with gold nanoparticles was developed to determine pork adulteration in beef and chicken meatball preparations.

Nanotechnology in Food Packaging

A recent challenge in the food packaging Industry is the concept called "smart packaging", wherein packaging is not a passive container, it provides additional functionality beyond containing, protecting, and supplying information about the food. Smart packaging is classified as "active" or "intelligent package." An active package is characterized by presence of active constituents that involves interaction of packaging material with food and environment. An intelligent package contains a device that monitors condition of the product, package, packaging environment and prevent counterfeiting. Sensing is an important part of intelligent packaging system. A shift towards inclusion of nanomaterials in existing packaging materials might help to improve properties of packaging materials. Nanoparticles can impart significant barrier properties, as well as mechanical, optical, catalytic, and antimicrobial properties into packaging. Basic properties of materials packaging like flexibility, durability, flame resistance, barrier and recycling properties can be modified with addition of nanomaterials. According to a report by Persistence Market Research in 2014, the global nano-enabled packaging market for food and beverages will be $15.0 billion in 2020.

Currently, a variety of nanomaterials have been introduced to food packaging as functional additives like silver nanoparticle , nanoclay, nano-zinc oxide, nano-titanium dioxide, carbon nanotubes , cellulose nano-whiskers, and starch nanocrystals. Due to differences in chemical structure and characteristics, each nanomaterial introduces distinct properties to the host material, for lead to different functional packaging applications. Silver nanoparticles and nanocomposites were the most widely used nanomaterials as antimicrobials in the food industry. A dozen silver-containing zeolites have been approved by the U.S. FDA for use as food contact materials for the purpose of disinfection.

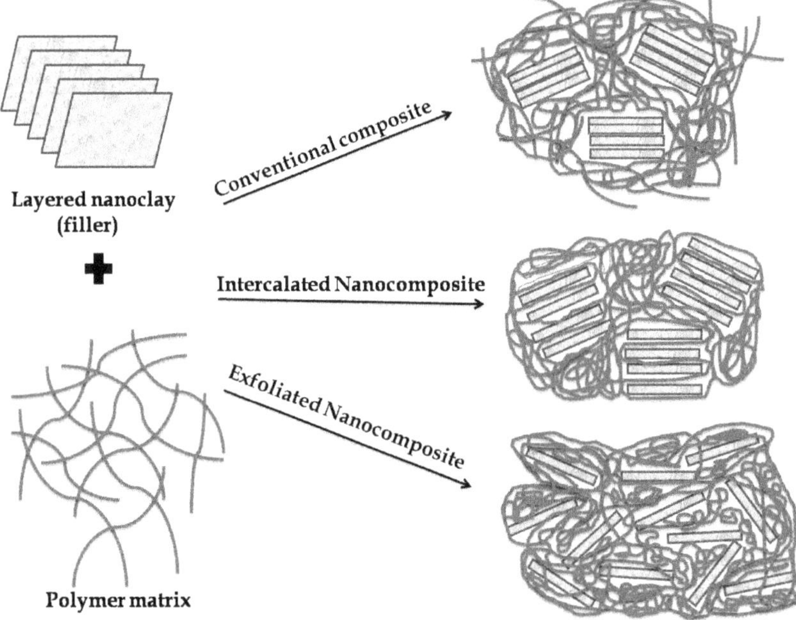

Fig. 2: Graphical representation on types of nanocomposites formed from polymer matrix and layered nanoclay (Credit: Haripriya Shanmugam and Preetha Sundharam)

Nanocomposites are materials that incorporate nanoparticles into the matrix of a standard packaging material. Polymers are largely engineered to form nanocomposites with metal/metal oxide nanoparticles for food application. Among these polymers, low-density polyethylene (LDPE), gelatin and isotactic polypropylene are most widely used as part of nanocomposites. However, environmentally sustainable biopolymers like polylactic acid (PLA), polycaprolactone (PCL), and poly (butylene succinate) (PBS) have become attractive materials for many food packaging applications. However, these biopolymers exhibit poor barrier with weak mechanical properties, so they are used as composite materials. Nanoclay has been recognized as major reinforcement filler for biopolymer. Very low clay content can improve barrier property, modulus, creep resistance, and mechanical strength of bio-polymer, while biodegradability remains intact. Among the polymer nanocomposites for food packaging, nanoclay was the first material to emerge to the market and today, it is the most widely used nanomaterial in food packaging. In the past, plastic bottles did not adequately retain the gas and the flavor of beer or soda, because of their poor gas barrier property. However, this challenge has been overcome by integrating nanoclay into the polymer matrix and is now extensively used for beverage packaging. Silver nanoparticles and nanoclay account for the majority of the nano-enabled food packaging in the market. In the market, these nanomaterials are primarily used to impart antimicrobial property and to improve barrier properties, thereby extending the shelf life and freshness of packaged food.

Fresh cut perishables (fruits and vegetables) and ready-to-eat foods are prone to surface contamination resulting in reduced shelf life. Edible coatings/films are formed by one or several thin layers of biopolymer based materials with specific functionality (antimicrobial property) that will become part of the food to be consumed. The film improves shelf life of the produce without any environmental pollution (no wastages). Proteins are desirable for the production of edible films or coatings, as it has better oxygen and water vapour barrier properties. Nanostructured edible films can improve the property of the films in prolonging shelf life as well as its antimicrobial property. However, there is a growing concern about migration of nanomaterials from food contact materials to food materials and its associated potential risks.

Food Labeling

Two dimensional barcodes are globally used as product authentication labels. But these barcodes can be easily traced and are prone to damage, alteration as well as falsification. Nanoparticle based invisible barcodes can be labeled without being noticed and are hard to manipulate. Invisible nanobarcode tags of 7400 unique barcodes have been reported. Fluorescent deoxyribonucleic acid dendrimer nanobarcodes have been reported for detection of *E. coli,* anthrax and tularemia, ebola and severe acute respiratory syndrome pathogens in food samples. Different nanobarcodes were assigned to each microorganism. Nanobarcode detection can be performed using fluorescent microscopy and radio-frequency identification (RFID) with ease.

Safety Concerns

According to an article published in the "Journal of food and drug analysis" (2016), studies have focused on the potential toxicity of presence of nanomaterials by analyzing food samples used in food additives/ingredients and food packaging. It infers that not much information is available on bioavailability, biodistribution space and ultimate toxicity upon exposure to them. Interestingly, increased usage of nanostructures incorporated food additives like flavour and colour that comes in direct contact with human organs have received significant attention from public and government sectors. This may result in higher levels of exposure depending on their concentration in food and the amount of food consumed. Increasing use of nanomaterials in lipid/protein-based nanoencapsulation food systems are also being developed to improve their solubility and bioavailability in humans. However, safety of nanoencapsulation remains uninvestigated and its risk assessment for long-term toxicity needs to be studied. Another case of exposure may occur unintentionally through leaching from nanopackaging. Nanoclay and edible nanofilms from food contact materials were found to migrate into the food stimulants. Inhalation of food packaging nanomaterials and their entrance through skin penetration is an occupational hazard for workers in food processing industries. It is inevitable that human exposure to nanomaterials in food systems will increase either intentionally or unintentionally in the near future. Currently, fate and potential toxicity of nanomaterials in food systems are not fully understood and there are significant advances in application of nanotechnology in the food industry. The associated health and environmental impacts should be analyzed and regulations should be framed. To be successful in the long run, proper education of the public is also necessary for introduction and development of nanotechnology based products with food systems.

Suggested Study Materials

1. Nanotechnology for food packaging and food quality assessment. 2017. M. Rossi, D. Passeri, A. Sinibaldi, M. Angjellari, E. Tamburri, A. Sorbo, E. Carata and L. Dini. Advances in Food and Nutrition Research ©Elsevier Inc.
2. Nanotechnology and functional foods : effective delivery of bioactive ingredients. 2015 . Edited by Cristina M. Sabliov, Hongda Chen, Rickey Y. Yada.© John Wiley & Sons, Ltd.
3. Techniques for nanoencapsulation of food ingredients. 2014. C. Anandharamakrishnan. Springer New York Heidelberg Dordrecht London.
4. Iris J. Joye, Gabriel Davidov-Pardo, David Julian McClements. 2014. Nanotechnology for increased micronutrient bioavailability. Trends in Food Science & Technology.

Self-assessment Questions

1. _______________ is the most widely used nanomaterial as antimicrobials in the food industry.
2. _______________ is a device that identifies specific volatile components of an odor in a food sample.
3. Nanoclay has been recognized as major reinforcement filler for biobased polymer. **True/False.**
4. Gold nanoparticles immobilised pyranose oxidase has been used for detection of glucose in fruit juices. **True/False**
5. What are all the advantages of nanoencapsulation of food bioactives?
6. How nanotechnology enhances oral bioavailability of bioactives?
7. Name two food bioactives with poor aqueous solubility?
8. Difference between active and intelligent packaging?
9. Write a note on nanoencapsulation of food bioactives with an example?
10. Write a detailed on note about safety issues associated with application of nanotechnology in food systems?

16

Application of Nanotechnology in Energy and Environment

Dr. S Marimuthu

The global energy demand is growing due to the population burst and forecasted to rise by 50 per cent by 2030. According to the forecast of International Energy Agency, the energy demand will rise from the current use of 12000 MTOE (Million Ton Oil Equivalent) to more than 18000 MTOE until 2030. Now, the primary energy demand is covered by fossil fuels, however, the oil reserve will be exhausted in couple of decades. The nuclear fuel covers part of the energy demand, which will be also short in the near future. In the view of post- climate change scenarios like rise in atmospheric carbon dioxide and decline in the fossil fuel reserve in the near future, it becomes clear that the energy demand will be satisfied through the increased use of renewable energy sources, which include sun, wind, tides, geothermy, batteries and plant biomass. The current levels of technologies in renewable energy sources are inefficient and expensive for the adoption. The Nanotechnology is the emerging field which offers solutions in wide spectrum of areas including the energy sector to develop and optimize processes for higher energy efficiency and economically viable. In this chapter, it will be discussed on the scope of nanotechnology in renewable sources of energy.

Solar Energy

Solar energy has huge potential to realize the energy demand in the future. India like tropical countries are blessed with solar radiation almost throughout the year, which amounts to 3,000 hours of sunshine @ 4-7 kWh of solar radiation per sq metres, which is equivalent to more than 5,000 trillion kWh.

Photovoltaic cells convert light into electrical energy. A French physicist, Edmund Becquerel, first observed the physical phenomenon responsible for converting light to electricity the photovoltaic effect in 1839. Photovoltaic cell is composed of a thin wafer consisting of an ultra-thin layer of phosphorus-doped (N-type) silicon on top of a thicker layer of boron-doped (P-type) silicon.

An electrical field is created near the top surface of the cell where these two materials are in contact, called the P-N junction. When sunlight hits panels, it results in the movement of electrons and holes. This electrical field provides momentum and direction to light-stimulated electrons, resulting in a flow of current when the solar panel is biased to an electrical load.

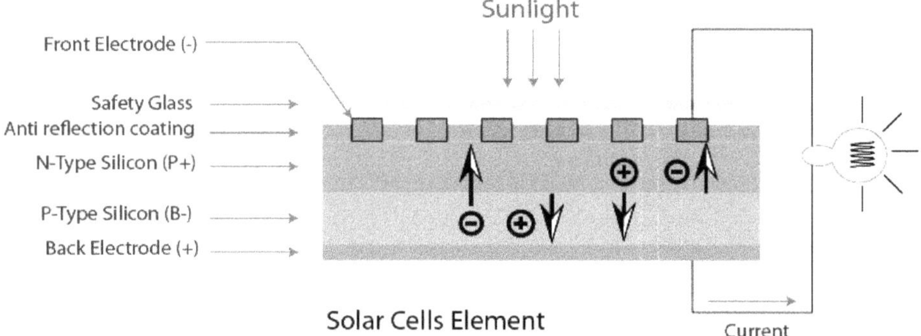

(Adopted from www.bestsale2u.com accessed on 20.09.2017)

Fig. 2: Illustration on components and working principle of photovoltaic cells

The current limitations of photovoltaic cells are cost and efficiency. The efficiency of light conversion in photovoltaic cells depends on the semiconductor, which is made up of solar panels. Semiconductors absorb sun light precisely with particular energy spectrum depends on its band gap and theoretically it works to be 33 per cent conversion efficiency for crystalline silicon panels. Practically it have reached only 11 per cent at maximum. Nanotechnology contributes to the improvement of Photovoltaic device efficiency.

Antireflective Coatings in Solar Panels

Increasing the amount of light that reaches the active light sensitive material will improve the efficiency of photovoltaic devices. Antireflection coatings dramatically reduce reflection losses, and light transmission is significantly improved by exploiting photonic crystals, plasmonic guiding and other nanoscale coupling structures. Silicon nanotips on solar panel cells, which are nanostructures mimicking moth's eye for anti reflective layers. Nano Titanium dioxide is the most widely for making antireflective surface using white pigment because of its brightness, high refractive index and excellent stability. Poly (Methyl Methacrylate) is another candidate for creating antireflective surface in the solar panels. The mechanism of anti-reflection coating follows Fresnel equation explains that there would be no reflection if there is a destructive interference between light reflected from the coating substrate and the air-coating interfaces.

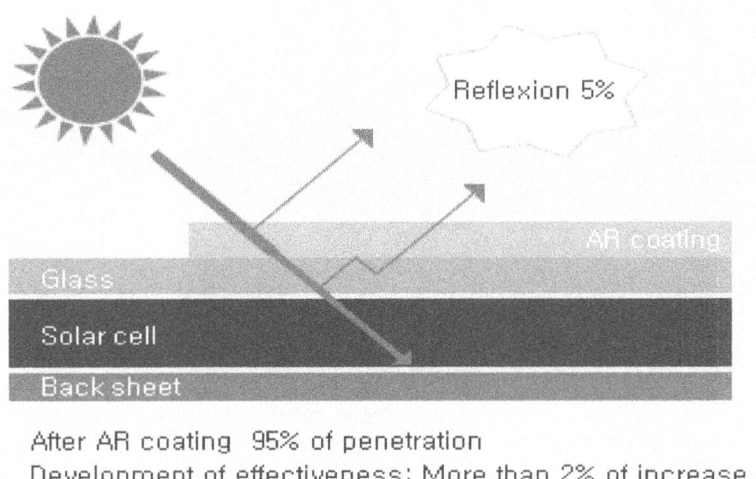

(Adopted from www.hyseoul.com accessed on 20.09.2017)

Fig. 2: AR refers to antireflective coating which improve transmission of light reducing refection from the surface

Self-cleaning Solar Panels

Solar panel conversion efficiency, typically in the 20 percent range, is reduced by dust, grime, pollen, and other particulates that accumulate on the solar panel. A dirty solar panel reduce its power capabilities by up to 30 per cent in high dust/ pollen or desert areas due to reduction in the transmission of light. Self-cleaning is a property which is explored for keep dust free solar panels. Wettability is an important property of a solid surface, and contact angle (θ) which are commonly used to characterize the surface hydrophilicity. The leaf of the lotus plant is a representative model for super hydrophobic and self-cleaning surface due to the presence of papillose epidermal cells covered with wax crystals. This makes water droplets on the surface are in the Cassie-Baxter state (Keeping water contact angle >150°), making them highly spherical and be able to roll off easily in the lotus leaf. The phenomenon is referred as Lotus effect. Usually, contaminants are larger than the cellular structure of the leaves, leaving the particles resting on the tips of papillae. When a water droplet rolls over the contaminants, it moves dirt particles from the surface by making them to adsorb with water droplets (Fig 3). Solar cells are coated with Zinc Oxide nanowire ad Titanium di oxide allows the surface of the solar cell to self-clean via photocatalytic degradation of organic material by high surface area and increase the water contact angle to super hydrophobic (>150°), resulting in self-cleaning of solar panels. Ethanolic suspension of perfluorosilane-coated titanium dioxide nanoparticles are also used for self-cleaning in solar panels.

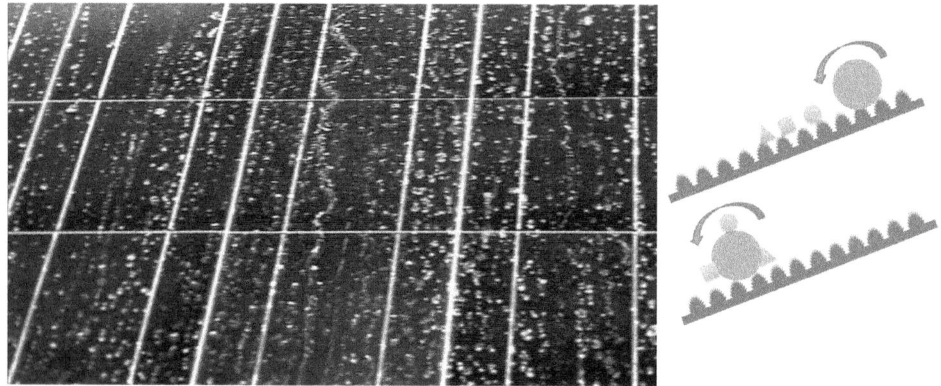

Fig. 3: Self-cleaning solar panels for dust free in panels (Courtesy: University of Houston) and mechanism of self-cleaning *(Courtesy: He, 2016, P.No 9)*

Tandem or Multi-Junction Solar Cells

Tandem solar cells are made of multiple materials with different bandgaps to capture a range of the solar spectrum. Unlike single solar cell, which absorbs specific spectrum of energy, tandem solar cells absorb wide range of solar spectrum due to the presence of materials with different band gaps. Hence tandem cell records higher photo conversion efficiency. Multi-junction solar cells structure is multi-layers of alloys from group III and V elements staked over each other in such a way that higher the band gap of the materials form the top layer in the solar cell (Fig 4).

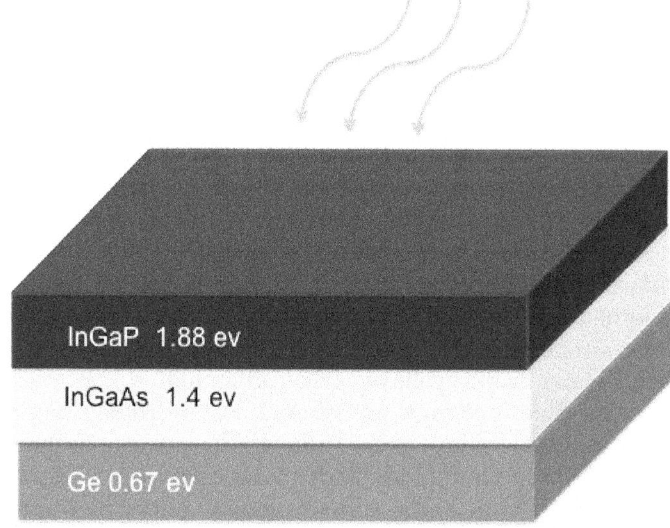

(Courtesy: Stanford University)

Fig. 4: Tandem solar cells of multiple materials with different band gaps

Solar cells with more junctions are fabricated such as an InGaP (Indium Gallium Phosphide/GaAs (Gallium Arsenide)/InGaAsN (Indium Gallium Arsenic Nitride/ Ge (Germanium) four-junction structure to improve photo conversion efficiency. Tandem solar cells made of III-V elements have advantage for tuning bandgap by elemental compositions in order to capture wide range of solar spectrum and achieve higher photon absorption and conversion efficiency. The energy balance calculation shows that the efficiency cannot exceed 31 per cent with single junction solar cell. The band gap of silicon is 1.1 eV, and hence, silicon's photo conversion efficiency is limited to 29 per cent. If tandem cell has two material layer tuned to bandgap of 1.64 eV while the other layer to 0.94 e respectively, it will provide a theoretical conversion performance of 44 per cent. Similarly, a three-layer cell can be tuned to a band gap of 1.83, 1.16 and 0.71 eV, to achieve the efficiency of 48 per cent. An "infinity-layer" cells would have a theoretical efficiency of 86 per cent.

Dye Sensitized Solar Cells

Dye-sensitized solar cells (DSSC) are thin-film photovoltaic cell invented in 1988 by Brian O'Regan and Michael Grätzel. Dye sensitized Solar cell is sandwich structure having conducting oxide electrodes filling the interlayer with organic redox electrolyte. Dye-sensitized solar cells are also referred as Gratzel cells. Mesoporous titanium oxide are deposited onto conducting electrodes. The exposure of solar cell to light energy leads to the excitation of organic dye (N3 ruthenium complex) ejecting electrons to the conduction band of titanium oxide semiconductors, which adsorbed over the dye. The electrons pass through the semiconductor layer reaches conducting oxide electrode (working electrode). The original state of the dye is restored by electron donation from the redox system, such as the iodide/triiodide couple. The regeneration of the organic dye by iodide intercepts absorbs photons get excited to release electron. The iodide is regenerated at the counter electrode received electron through the external load. The cycle continues to generate electrical energy, absorbing solar energy by organic dye molecules. Dye sensitized solar cells are regarded as third-generation solar technology capturing more sunlight per unit surface area. The solar cells are highly suitable under diffused sun light and cloudy skies. The technology is economical made out of stable resource materials and suitable for low density applications. It plays significant role in portable electronics and house hold applications

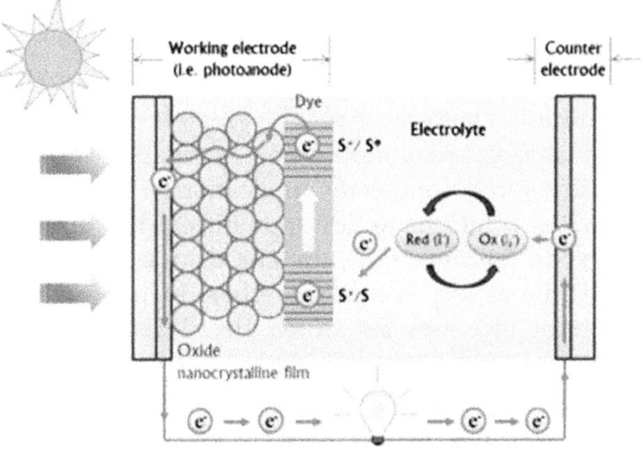

(Adopted from Alagarsamy et al., 2016)

Fig. 5: Illustration on the working of dye sensitized solar cells

Wind Energy

Wind energy is the low cost, emission free and clean one among the alternate energy sources. India is the fourth largest country in terms of wind power generation. Still power generated form wind turbines are costly than conventional resources. There are issues wind industry in terms of turbine performance, reliability for longer time, fatigue failure and cost of generation. The nanotechnologies such as nanoparticle-containing lubricants to remove fatigue, nanocoatings for de-icing and self-cleaning, and nanocomposites for lighter and stronger wind blades

The cost of rotor blades, gearbox and tower accounts for 50 60 per cent of the wind turbine installation. Tribo-corrosion (the degradation process of the material) and micro pitting of the rotating parts are the most important mechanisms for the damage of the structural components in wind turbines. Nanocomposite lubricants made from Molybdenum disulphide nanoparticles provide advanced boundary layer lubrication, which reduce friction and wear in turbines. Nano lubricants use the geometrical structure of nano particles, which behave like mini ball bearings, to provide extraordinary anti-wear and protection.

Advanced nanocoatings for de-icing and self-cleaning improve efficiencies of wind turbines preventing ice and dirt buildup on the blades. Coating of Carbon Nano-Tubes over the rotor blades and biasing with small electric current (carbon nano tube is super conductor of electricity) heats up rotor blades and prevents ice formation over the blades.

Larger wind turbines capture more wind energy however, which are hindered by the weight of blades. The heavier the blades, the more wind is needed to turn the rotor results in capturing less energy and hence wind turbine industry needs lighter and stiffer blades for harvesting maximum energy. Rotor blades made up of polyurethane blade reinforced with carbon nanotubes provide lighter and substantially stronger blades, which are having more than five times the tensile strength of carbon fiber and more than 60 times that of aluminum.

Lithium Batteries

Lithium-ion batteries have the greatest power density per unit weight and hence it revolutionized portable electronics. Still rechargeable batteries require higher density storage for specific applications with much higher life span. Nanotechnology provides solutions to develop efficient lithium batteries with higher density and life span. Lithium ions are stored in anode electrodes in rechargeable batteries when the battery is charged, where increasing the number of stored lithium ions in anode increases the stored electrical power. Electrodes made from nanoscale materials play a key role in the development of high-density batteries. Coating the electrode's surface with nanoparticles, nanowires, or other nanostructures provides more surface area for absorbing lithium ions. Electrode with carbon nanofibers in the lithium- ion battery showed four times higher storage capacity than the level of current lithium ion batteries. Similarly, changing elements in the electrode for attaching lithium ions also improves the performance of battery.

Sulfur is promising cathode materials for lithium batteries owing to its high specific capacity. Sulfur – titanium dioxide yolk–shell nanoarchitectures, polymer-encapsulated hollow sulfur nanospheres, carbon nanofibers encapsulating the sulfur are used as cathodes materials in lithium batteries for improving the charge density.

Fuel Cells

Fuel cell is next generation clean energy, electrochemical device, which converts hydrogen and oxygen into electricity through electro catalytic process. Fuel cell consists of an anode and a cathode filled with polymer electrolyte membrane, which acts as an ion carrier. Hydrogen is used as fuel fed to the anode where it is spilt into electrons and protons. Electrons are moved through an external circuit and reach the cathode while protons cross through polymer membrane electrolyte. Electrons and protons are combined together with oxygen in the cathode to produce water **(Fig 6).**

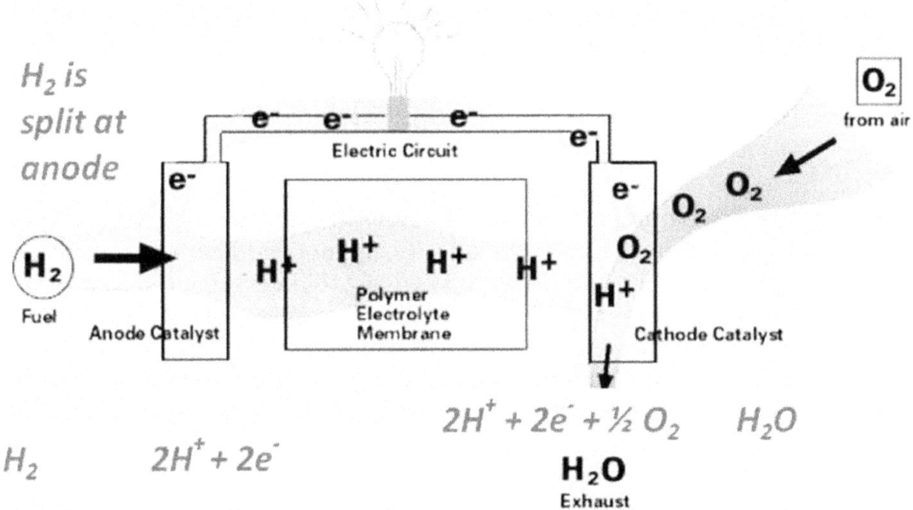

Fig 6: Fuel cells consists of cathode and anode separated with polymer electrolyte membrane where hydrogen is split at anode through electro oxidation releasing electrons and protons reaching cathode where both combines with oxygen to form water

Nanotechnologies provide scope for optimization of electrodes, proton membrane, and catalysts to improve the performance of fuel cells. Reduced catalytic activity is the common issue in the anode. Generally, carbon monoxide is a by-product during hydrogen production reactions in the anode chamber. The presence of carbon monoxide reduces catalytic activity at the anode due to chemisorption nature of carbon monoxide. The phenomenon is known as carbon monoxide poisoning ion fuel cells. Platinum/ruthenium-based nanocomposite is used as catalyst instead of platinum alone for improving catalytic activity avoiding the poisoning of carbon monoxide in anode chamber. Similarly one dimensional platinum nano rods/nano wires improve catalytic activity because of higher surface area in nano structured platinum. The catalytic activity is directly proportional with surface area of the catalyst. Three dimensional platinum–cobalt nanowire assemblies promote fuel cell activity. Higher Oxygen Reduction rates are higher in porous platinum nanotubes and nanoporous alloys such as Platinum Nickel and Platinum Nickel Aluminum alloys, It is established that higher porosity is achieved in nanostructure catalysts of size less than 15 nm. Swelling, fuel cross over, ionic (proton) conduction which requires humidity, operation of membrane in the limited range of temperature are the common limitations associated with polymer membrane electrolyte. Higher proton conductivity is reported in an electrolyte composed of carbon nano tube and sulfonated poly (ether ether ketone). Nano- composite membrane Polyphenylsulfone nanofibers reinforcing perfluorosulfonic acid improved proton conductivity and showed less dependence oh humidity for proton conduction. Recently electro spinning is employed to fabricate nano-membrane for improving the proton conduction and reduce the crossover of other contaminants.

Nano porous silica layer over polymer membrane electrolyte ensures water stays in the nanopores, which in turn combines with the acid molecules along the wall of the nanopores to form an acidic solution, This provide an easy pathway for hydrogen ions to move through the membrane, recording 100 times better conductivity of hydrogen ions than that of currently existing membrane.

Biofuels

Plant biomass is the largest primary resource for satisfying future fuel requirements with zero net emission of carbon dioxide. Bioethanol and biodiesel are currently in use to replace gasoline and diesel respectively. Biodiesel is produced through transesterification process from oils with an acid or base catalyst. Enzyme-based technologies are becoming popular for extracting biodiesel however the process suffer from low enzyme activity, high cost, poor catalysts recovery, and more range of operation for temperature. Nanoscale materials offer higher surface area for enzyme loading compared to bulk materials and increase the diffusion rate of substrates to the enzymes, thereby improving the rate of conversion into biodiesel. Lipase enzyme was immobilized in polyvinyl alcohol nanofibrous membranes and silver nanoparticles exhibited superior activity than that of local crude enzymes. Nano immobilized enzymes showed better temperature tolerance during the reaction. Reusability of immobilized lipase in silver nano particles are better than crude enzyme complex. Calcium oxide nano crystals with crystallite size of 20 nm gave 99 per cent conversion of soybean oil to biodiesel. Catalyst in nano structures are used are used to improve the rate of reaction and yield.

The ethanol produced typically has residual moisture content of ~ 4–6 percent and removal of this water by distillation is an energy-intensive process but the hydrophilic zeolites offer a low-energy intensive and cost effective option with improved ability in selectively removing water from ethanol.. The high silicon and aluminum composition in zeolites have selective affinity for more hydrophobic fuels where, selectivity for ethanol over water range from 10 and 100 for zeolites.

Power Transmission

Copper-based grids leak electricity at about 5 percent for 100 miles of transmission. whereas carbon nanotubes, (armchair) grids exhibit extraordinarily low electrical resistance (10 times better conductivity than copper) and tremendous specific tensile strength proved less loss of power during transmission useful in making power supply line in high-voltage grids.

High-temperature superconductors made with yttrium-barium copper oxide on metallic carriers proved highly efficient for low-loss wired power supply, has wide application in coil windings and bearings of electric engines. Power electronics ensure low loss power conversion in sub -sea cables which run for longer distances semiconductors where materials with high band gap, like silicon carbide are proposed for the application.

To summarize the chapter, sustainable energy production in future depends on the renewable sources where nanotechnology finds huge role to play during the production and processing of fuels besides its significance role in power transmission and storage.

Self-assessment Questions

Fill in the blanks

1. ____________ dye used in the Dye sensitized solar cells as photo sensitizer
2. ______________________ is used for long distance transmission of power instead of copper.
3. ______________________ invented dye sensitized solar cells
4. __________________, catalyst used in the electro oxidation of hydrogen in the fuel cells
5. The nanomaterial used in the self cleaning solar panels is ____________

Short answers

1. Define tandem solar cells
2. Define photovoltaic effect
3. Illustrate working principle of solar cells
4. What are the advantages of Dye Sensitized Solar cells?
5. Name the nanomaterials used for anti reflective coating in solar cells.
6. Define Gratzel cell
7. Describe the role of nanotechnology in the development of solar cells and wind turbines
8. Illustrate the working principle of fuel cells
9. Describe the role of nanotechnology in energy systems
10. List out any two applications of nanotechnology in the development of rechargeable batteries

17

Applications in Health Sciences and Nanotoxicology

Dr K S Subramanian & Dr S K Rajkishore

The characterization of the potential health impact of engineered materials produced through nanotechnology is an emerging issue of considerable discussion and debate. The current focus on nanotoxicity fails to assess the risk in different local environments and populations. People in developing countries may be more prone to adverse effects of nanoparticles because of underlying health conditions and malnutrition. Moreover, genetic susceptibility to toxic effects varies in diverse ethnic groups and geographical areas. The scientific community needs to identify these information gaps before developing regulations and standard methodologies for nanotoxicity assessment.

The skin is the largest organ of the body and serves as a primary route of environmental and/or occupational exposure; it is one of the principal portals of entry by which environmental toxicants or nanomaterials can enter into the body. At present, there is no information on whether nanoparticles can be absorbed across the stratum corneum barrier or whether systemically administered particles can accumulate in dermal tissue. Skin is unique because it provides an environment within the avascular epidermis where particles could potentially lodge and not be susceptible to removal by phagocytosis. The ability for nanomaterials to traverse the skin is a primary determinant of their dermatotoxic potential.

One of the major decisions to be faced in assessing the skin absorption and toxicity of nanomaterials is how to conduct the experiments. Should in vitro cell cultures, flow-through diffusion cells or cell lines be used? In vivo studies conducted in rat or preferably pig skin (since it is anatomically, physiologically, and biochemically similar to man) would be ideal. However, there are limitations in obtaining the quantity and quality of some nanomaterials to conduct in vivo studies. Therefore, in some cases it may be best to study their interactions in vitro in order to estimate the in vivo starting dose for toxicity. In vitro studies have shown that multi-walled carbon nanotubes (not derivatized or optimized for biological applications) are capable of localizing within and initiating an irritation response in human epidermal keratinocytes, which are a primary route of occupational exposure.

A systematic tier approach can be implemented for evaluating nanomaterials. In vitro testing, followed by escalation to more complex testing models, may render useful information in the evaluation of these materials in lieu of chronic bioassays. Short-term mechanistic studies, in vitro studies, and ultra fine particle epidemiological studies can provide important enhancements to traditional toxicity assays. Integrating this information increases our confidence in the hazard identification of nanoparticles, and when coupled with exposure considerations, the risk assessment of nanomaterials.

Determination of the mode of action (MOA) for effects observed with nanomaterials will be a key issue in understanding data obtained from toxicological evaluations and its extrapolation for the determination of potential human health risk. Some of the key MOA considerations for nanoscale materials include: (1) do their unique physicochemical properties translate into unique MOAs?; (2) what are the best experimental strategies to obtain data that can identify key events with which to evaluate these MOAs?; (3) can evaluation of a core set of parameters and/or model materials be used to determine MOAs that can be applied to emerging nanomaterials?

Nanomaterials cannot simply be considered as a single homogeneous class. In addition, our current understanding of the MOA of nanomaterials is very limited, since research to date has only been conducted on a few example materials. There are a number of parameters that will be key to understanding the MOA for a given material, including the size/shape/aspect ratio, hardness/deformability, composition, surface area and surface chemistry, types of coatings/modifications and stability. Given that nanomaterials vary greatly based on these parameters, extrapolation of a MOA from one material to another will need to be made with extreme caution until more knowledge is gained on a broader class of materials. A number of studies have documented *in vitro* and *in vivo* toxicity of exposure to nanoparticles. Evidence suggests they can induce DNA damage, reactive oxygen species, damage to cellular organelles and cell death. This necessitates the requirement of Biosafety studies to be performed while developing any products with nanoparticles.

Nano-toxicities

- The rapidly developing field of nanotechnology is likely to become yet another source for human exposures to NSPs—engineered nanoparticles (NPs)—by different routes: inhalation (respiratory tract), ingestion [gastrointestinal (GI) tract], dermal (skin), and injection (blood circulation). Table 1 summarizes some of the natural and anthropogenic sources of NSPs, the latter divided into unintentional and intentional sources.

- Biologically based or naturally occurring molecules that are found inside organisms since the beginning of life can serve as model nanosized materials. A biologic model of coated nanomaterials can be found in ferritin, which is an approximately 12-nm-large iron storage protein that contains 5- to 7-nm-sized hydrous ferric oxide phosphate inside a protective protein shell. Nanosized materials, including fullerenes, occur naturally from combustion processes such as forest fires and volcanoes.
- Obvious differences between unintentional and intentional anthropogenic NSPs are the polydispersed and chemically complex nature (elemental, soluble, and volatile carbon compounds; soluble and poorly soluble inorganics of the former, in contrast to the monodisperse and precise chemically engineered characteristics and solid form of the latter, generated in gas or liquid phase [National Nanotechnology Initiative (NNI) 2004].
- The extraordinarily high number concentrations of NSPs per given mass will likely be of toxicologic significance when these particles interact with cells and subcellular components. Likewise, their increased surface area per unit mass can be toxicologically important if other characteristics such as surface chemistry and bulk chemistry are the same. Although the mass of UFPs in ambient air is very low, approaching only 0.5–2 $\mu g/m^3$ at background levels and it can increase several-fold during high pollution episodes or on highways.

Physicochemical Characteristics as Determinants of Biologic Activity

- The small size and corresponding large specific surface area of solid NSPs confer specific properties to them, for example, making them desirable as catalysts for chemical reactions. The importance of surface area becomes evident when considering that surface atoms or molecules play a dominant role in determining bulk properties; the ratio of surface to total atoms or molecules increases exponentially with decreasing particle size. Increased surface reactivity predicts that NSPs exhibit greater biologic activity per given mass compared with larger particles, should they be taken up into living organisms and provided they are solid rather than solute particles. This increased biologic activity can be either positive and desirable (e.g., antioxidant activity, carrier capacity for therapeutics, penetration of cellular barriers for drug delivery) or negative and undesirable (e.g., toxicity, induction of oxidative stress or of cellular dysfunction), or a mix of both.
- The characteristic biokinetic behaviors of NPs are attractive qualities for promising applications in medicine as diagnostic and therapeutic devices and as tools to investigate and understand molecular processes and structures in living cells. For example, targeted drug delivery to tissues that are difficult to reach [e.g., central nervous system (CNS)], NPs for the fight against cancer, intra-vascular nanosensor and nanorobotic devices, and diagnostic and imaging procedures are presently under development.

The discipline of nanomedicine—defined as medical application of nanotechnology and related research—has arisen to design, test, and optimize these applications so that they can eventually be used routinely by physicians.

Human Exposure to Nanosized Materials

- In addition to natural and anthropogenic sources of UFPs in the ambient air, certain workplace conditions also generate NSPs that can reach much higher exposure concentrations, up to several hundred micrograms per cubic meter, than is typically found at ambient levels. Inhalation may be the major route of exposure for NPs, yet ingestion and dermal exposures also need to be considered during manufacture, use, and disposal of engineered nanomaterials, and specific biomedical applications for diagnostic and therapeutic purposes will require intravenous, subcutaneous, or intramuscular administration. Manufactured nanomaterials in the environment.

Toxicology of Airborne UFPs

- In recent years, interest in potential effects of exposure to airborne UFPs has increased considerably, and studies have shown that they can contribute to adverse health effects in the respiratory tract as well as in extrapulmonary organs. Results on direct effects of ambient and model UFPs have been reported from epidemiologic studies and controlled clinical studies in humans, inhalation/instillation studies in rodents, or in vitro cell culture systems. For example, several epidemiologic studies have found associations of ambient UFPs with adverse respiratory and cardiovascular effects resulting in morbidity and mortality in susceptible parts of the population.
- In vitro studies using different cell systems showed varying degrees of proinflammatory-and oxidative-stress–related cellular responses after dosing with laboratory-generated or filter-collected ambient UFPs. Collectively, the in vitro results have identified oxidative-stress–related changes of gene expression and cell signaling pathways as underlying mechanisms of UFP effects, as well as a role of transition metals and certain organic compounds on combustion-generated UFPs Concepts of Nanotoxicology Top

Reactive Oxygen Species Mechanisms of NSP Toxicity

- Both in vivo and in vitro, NSPs of various chemistries have been shown to create reactive oxygen species (ROS). ROS production has been found in NPs as diverse as C60 fullerenes, SWNTs, quantum dots, and UFPs, especially under concomitant exposure to light, UV, or transition metals. It has been demonstrated that NSPs of various sizes and various chemical compositions preferentially mobilize to mitochondria. Because mitochondria are redox active organelles, there is a likelihood of altering

ROS production and thereby overloading or interfering with antioxidant defenses.

- The exact mechanism by which each of these diverse NPs cause ROS is not yet fully understood, but suggested mechanisms include a) photo excitation of fullerenes and SWNTs, causing intersystem crossing to create free electrons; b) metabolism of NPs to create redox active intermediates, especially if metabolism is via cytochrome P450s; and c) inflammation responses in vivo that may cause oxyradical release by macrophages. Other mechanisms will likely emerge as studies on NP toxicity continue.
- The small size and respective large specific surface area of NPs, like those of ambient airborne UFPs, give them unique properties with respect to a potential to cause adverse effects. Certainly, as shown in studies with UFPs, chemical composition and other particle parameters are additional important effect modifiers. Results from these studies will therefore serve as a basis for future studies in the field of nanotoxicology, for example, the propensity of NSPs to translocate across cell layers and along neuronal pathways (see "Disposition of NSPs in the respiratory tract" below).

Portals of Entry and Target Tissues

- Most of the toxicity research on NSPs in vivo has been carried out in mammalian systems, with a focus on respiratory system exposures for testing the hypothesis that airborne UFPs cause significant health effects. With respect to NPs, other exposure routes, such as skin and GI tract, also need to be considered as potential portals of entry. Portal-of-entry–specific defense mechanisms protect the mammalian organism from harmful materials. However, these defenses may not always be as effective for NSPs, as is discussed below.

Respiratory Tract

- In order to appreciate what dose the organism receives when airborne particles are inhaled, information about their deposition as well as their subsequent fate is needed. Here we focus on the fate of inhaled nanosized materials both within the respiratory tract itself and translocated out of the respiratory tract. There are significant differences between NSPs and larger particles regarding their behaviour during deposition and clearance in the respiratory tract.

Disposition of NSPs in the Respiratory Tract

- Once deposited, NSPs—in contrast to larger-sized particles—appear to translocate readily to extrapulmonary sites and reach other target organs by different transfer routes and mechanisms. One involves transcytosis across epithelia of the respiratory tract into the interstitium and access to the blood circulation directly or via lymphatics, resulting in distribution throughout the body. The other is a not generally recognized mechanism that appears to be distinct for NSPs and that involves their uptake by sensory nerve endings embedded in airway epithelia, followed by axonal translocation to ganglionic and CNS structures.

Epithelial Translocation

- Because of the apparent inefficiency of alveolar macrophage phagocytosis of NSPs, one might expect that these particles interact instead with epithelial cells. Indeed, results from several studies show that NSPs deposited in the respiratory tract readily gain access to epithelial and interstitial sites. This was also shown in studies with ultrafine PTFE fumes: shortly after a 15-min exposure, the fluorine-containing particles could be found in interstitial and submucosal sites of the conducting airways as well as in the interstitium of the lung periphery close to the pleura. Such interstitial translocation represents a shift in target site away from the alveolar space to the interstitium, potentially causing direct particle-induced effects there.

Translocation to the Circulatory System

- Once the particles have reached pulmonary interstitial sites, uptake into the blood circulation, in addition to lymphatic pathways, can occur; again, this pathway is dependent on particle size, favoring NSPs. Within 30 min post exposure, they found large amounts of these particles in platelets of pulmonary capillaries; the researchers suggested that this is an elimination pathway for inhaled particles that is significant for transporting the smallest air pollutant particles—in particular, particles of tobacco smoke—to distant organs. They also hypothesized that this "might predispose to platelet aggregation with formation of microthrombi atheromatous plaques" (Berry *et al.* 1977).

Exposure via Skin

- A potentially important uptake route is through dermal exposure. The epidermis, consisting of the outer horny layer (stratum corneum), the prickle cell layer (stratum spinosum), and basal cell layer (stratum basale), forms a very tight protective layer for the underlying dermis. The dermis has a rich supply of blood and tissue macrophages, lymph vessels, dendritic cells (Langerhans, also in stratum spinosum of epidermis), and five different types of sensory nerve endings. Broken skin represents a readily available portal of entry even for larger (0.5–7 μm) particles, as evidenced by reports about accumulation of large amounts of soil particles in inguinal lymph nodes of people who often run or walk barefoot; this can be associated with elephantiatic lymphedema

Risk Assessment

- The lack of toxicology data on engineered NPs does not allow for adequate risk assessment. Because of this, some may even believe that engineered

NPs are so risky that they call for a precautionary halt in NP-related research. However, the precautionary principle should not be used to stop research related to nanotechnology and NPs. Instead, we should strive for a sound balance between further development of nanotechnology and the necessary research to identify potential hazards in order to develop a scientifically defensible database for the purpose of risk assessment. To be able to do this, a basic knowledge about mammalian and ecotoxicologic profiles of NPs is necessary, rather than attempting to assess NP risks based on some popular science fiction literature.

- Most important, sufficient resources should be allocated by governmental agencies and industries to be able to perform a scientifically based risk assessment and then establish justifiable procedures for risk management. The data needed for this risk assessment should be determined a priori so that limited resources can be used efficiently to develop useful and well-planned studies.

Summary

- Research on ambient UFPs has laid the foundation for the emerging field of nanotoxicology, with the goal of studying the biokinetics and the potential of engineered nanomaterials (particles, tubes, shells, quantum dots, etc.) to cause adverse effects.
- Major differences between ambient UFPs and NPs are the polydisperse nature of the former versus the monodisperse size of the latter, and particle morphology, oftentimes a branched structure from combustion particles versus spherical form of NPs, although other shapes (tubes, wires, rings, planes) are also manufactured. In addition, combustion-derived volatile organic compounds and inorganic constituents (e.g., metals, nitrates, sulfates) of different solubilities on UFPs predict differences in the toxicologic profile between UFPs and NPs. However, as far as the insoluble particle is concerned, concepts of NSPs kinetics, including cell interactions, will most likely be the same for UFPs and NPs.
- The introduction of nanostructured materials for biomedical and electronics applications opens tremendous opportunities for biomedical applications as therapeutic and diagnostic tools as well as in the fields of engineering, electronics, optics, consumer products, alternative energy, soil/water remediation, and others. However, very little is yet known about their potential to cause adverse effects or humoral immune responses once they are introduced into the organism—unintentionally or intentionally. Nanomedicine products will be well tested before introduction into the marketplace. However, for the manufacturers of most current nanotechnology products, regulations requiring nanomaterial-specific data on toxicity before introduction into the marketplace are an evolving area and presently under discussion (Bergeson and Auerbach 2004; Foresight and Governance Project 2003). During a product's life

cycle (manufacture, use, disposal), it is probable that nanomaterials will enter the environment, and currently there is no unified plan to examine ecotoxicologic effects of NPs. In addition, the stability of coatings and covalent surface modifications need to be determined both in ecologic settings and *in vivo*.

- Results of older biokinetic studies and some new toxicology studies with NSPs (mostly ambient UFPs) can be viewed as the basis for the expanding field of nanotoxicology. These studies showed that the greater surface area per mass renders NSPs more active biologically than larger-sized particles of the same chemistry, and that particle surface area and number appear to be better predictors for NSPs-induced inflammatory and oxidative stress responses. The following emerging concepts of nanotoxicology can be identified from these studies:
- The biokinetics of NSPs are different from larger particles. When inhaled, they are efficiently deposited in all regions of the respiratory tract; they evade specific defense mechanisms; and they can translocate out of the respiratory tract via different pathways and mechanisms (endocytosis and transcytosis). When in contact with skin, there is evidence of penetration to the dermis followed by translocation via lymph to regional lymph nodes. A possible uptake into sensory nerves needs to be investigated. When ingested, systemic uptake via lymph into the organism can occur, but most are excreted via feces. When in blood circulation, they can distribute throughout the organism, and they are taken up into liver, spleen, bone marrow, heart, and other organs. In general, translocation rates are largely unknown; they are probably very low but are likely to change in a compromised/diseased state.
- The biologic activity and biokinetics are dependent on many parameters: size, shape, chemistry, crystallinity, surface properties (area, porosity, charge, surface modifications, weathering of coating), agglomeration state, biopersistence, and dose. These parameters are likely to modify responses and cell interactions, such as a greater inflammatory potential than larger particles per given mass, translocation across epithelia from portal of entry to other organs, translocation along axons and dendrites of neurons, induction of oxidative stress, pro-oxidant and antioxidant activity of NSPs in environmentally relevant species, binding to proteins and receptors, and localization in mitochondria.
- The principles of cellular and organismal interactions discussed in this article should be applicable for both ambient UFPs and NPs, even if the latter are coated with a bio-compatible material. Knowledge about the bio-persistence of this coating is as essential as is knowledge about the bioavailability of the core material that could have intrinsic toxic properties, for example, semiconductor metal compounds in sub-10-nm quantum dots consisting of cadmium and lead compounds. The very small size of these materials makes them available to the same translocation processes

described here for polydisperse NSPs, possibly even in a more efficient way because of their uniform size. When studying biologic / toxicologic effects, new processes of interactions with subcellular structures (e.g., microtubuli, mitochondria) will likely be discovered.

- The diversity of engineered nanomaterials and of the potential effects represents major challenges and research needs for nanotoxicology, including also the need for assessing human exposure during manufacture and use. The goal to exploit positive aspects of engineered nanomaterials and avoid potential toxic effects can best be achieved through a multidisciplinary team effort involving researchers in toxicology, materials science, medicine, molecular biology, bioinformatics, and their subspecialties

Assays used for Nanotoxicity

Importance of invitro tests: The predictive value of in vitro cytotoxicity tests is based on the idea of 'basal' cytotoxicity – that toxic chemicals affect basic functions of cells which are common to all cells and that the toxicity can be measured by assessing cellular damage. The development of *in vitro* cytotoxicity assays has been driven by the need to limit animal experimentation whenever possible and to carry out tests with small quantities of compounds.

In vitro Test Models and Assays

Test models; as nanoparticles are known to cause toxicity through inhalation, dermal integration and in some cases by metabolism, lung cell lines (MRC-5,), epithelial cell line (HeLa, A549) and liver cell line (HepG2) will be generally used. Depending on the applicability and area of environmental exposure biosafety studies can be supplemented with specific cell lines and tissue as the product warrants.

Assays: Cell health can be monitored by numerous methods. Plasma membrane integrity, DNA synthesis, DNA content, enzyme activity, presence of ATP, and cellular reducing conditions are known indicators of cell viability and cell death.

There are three major categories of assays which will help in evaluating the toxicity of nano particles in *in vitro* system.

1. Cytotoxic assays (which mainly focus on cell viability, plasma membrane integrity and cellular metabolism).
2. Genotoxicity assays (which study the DNA structure breakage, mutagenicity, Chromosomal aberration etc.)
3. Alteration in gene expression assays

1. Cytotoxicity Assays

Any cytotoxic agent acting through the cell impacts the basic cellular metabolism. To study the basic cellular metabolism, the response of cell to any toxic agent is measured by the enzymes present on the cellular surface. This, in turn, reflects the changes in cell proliferation. There are many assays to study the intactness of cell and cellular metabolism which are described below:

1.1. Trypan Blue Exclusion Assay

In this assay cells are treated with agents, trypsinized, and subsequently stained with trypan blue, a diazo dye which is taken up by dead cells, but excluded by viable cells. Unstained cells reflect the total number of viable cells recovered from a given dish. This method is advantageous because it conveys the actual number of viable cells and increases (cell proliferation) or decreases (cytotoxicity) in comparison to control, untreated cells.

1.2. *In Vitro* Cell Viability Assay

Cell proliferation is quantified by WST-1/ MTT/ XTT reagent. This assay is by far the most sensitive and convenient method for quantifying cell proliferation and viability.The first assay type is the measurement of cellular metabolic activity. An early indication of cellular damage is a reduction in metabolic activity. Tests which can measure metabolic function measure cellular ATP levels or mitochondrial activity (via MTS metabolism). Mitochondrial activity is measured by this assay.

Principle: This is a colorimetric assay for the quantification of cell viability and proliferation. The enzyme succinate tetrazolium reductase cleaves tetrazolium salts (WST1) to formazan that is colored product and can be quantitatively measured in spectrophotometer at 450 nm. This enzyme belongs to the respiratory chain of the mitochondria and is active only in viable cells. The amount of formazan dye produced directly correlates the number of metabolically active cells.

1.3 Cytotoxicity Assay (LDH Assay)

Another parameter often tested is the measurement of membrane integrity. The cell membrane forms a functional barrier around the cell, and traffic into and out of the cell is highly regulated by transporters, receptors and secretion pathways. When cells are damaged, they become 'leaky' and this forms the basis for the second type of assay. Membrane integrity is determined by measuring lactate dehyrogenase (LDH) in the extra cellular medium. This enzyme is normally present in the cytosol, and cannot be measured extracellularly unless cell damage has occurred. It has been shown that changes in metabolic activity are better indicators of early cell injury and that effects on membrane integrity are indicative of more serious injury, leading to cell death. The enzyme lactate dehydrogenase (LDH-L) is distributed in all cells. Several colorimetric LDH-L assay methods have been developed. Most of these assays are based on the coupling of the reduction of NAD and tetrazolium salts (INT). Nachlas, *et al*, described an LDH-L assay using phenazine methosulfate (PMS) as the intermediate electron carrier between NADH and INT. Allain, *et al*, replaced PMS with the enzyme diaphorase.

Principle; The assay is based on the cleavage of a tetrazolium salt when LDH is present in the culture supernatant. The procedure involves incubating the cells

with any cytotoxic agent in culture may result in cell death. An increase in the amount of dead or plasma membrane-damaged cells during the assay results in an increase of LDH in the culture supernatant.

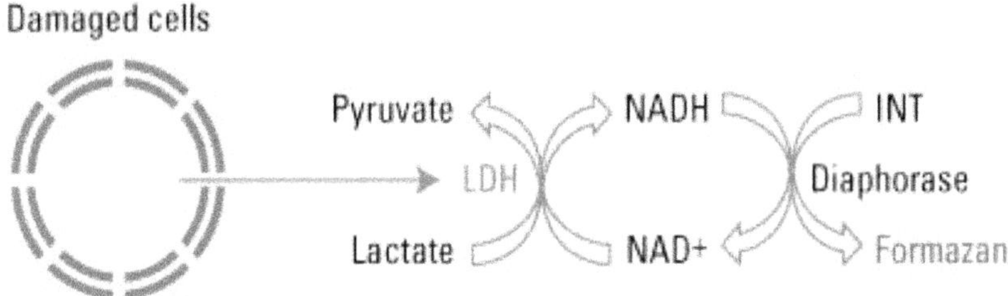

LDH catalyzes the oxidation of lactate to pyruvate in the presence of NAD which is subsequently reduced to NADH. The formation of NADH is coupled with the reduction of INT to INTH catalyzed by the enzyme of diaphorase. INTH is bright red formazan which is measured photo metrically at 500 ± 5 nm. The color intensity is proportional to the LDH-L activity of the sample.

2. Genotoxicity Assays

Generation of DNA damage is considered to be an important initial event in carcinogenesis. A considerable battery of assays exists for the detection of different genotoxic effects of compounds in experimental systems, or for investigations of exposure to genotoxic agents in environmental or occupational settings. The nanoparticles have been shown to be generating free radicals and these are highly reactive with DNA. Oxidative damage in DNA has often been suggested as a contributing factor in the process of aging and the development of cancer. There are many assays which can be employed to study the genotoxic potential of the Nanoparticles, which are described below.

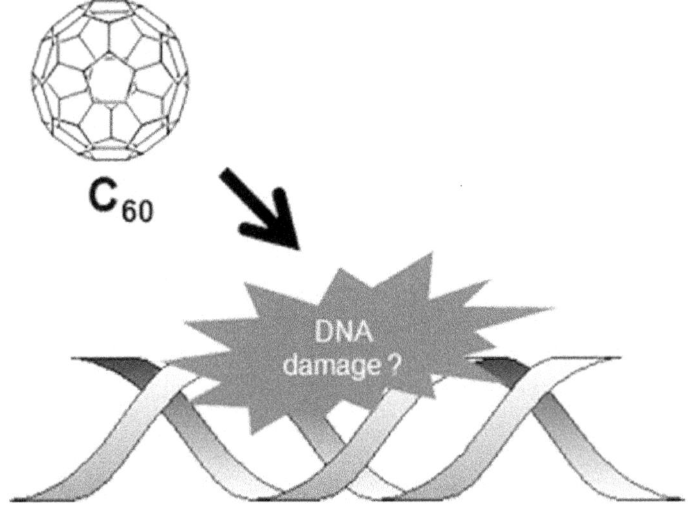

2.1 Determination of Gene Mutations Using the Ames Assay in *Salmonella typhimurium* and *Escherichia coli*

The reverse mutation (Ames) assay in *Salmonella typhimurium* employs bacteria deficient in DNA repair mechanisms that are unable to grow in the absence of histidine. Following exposure to compounds of interest, reversion to a histidine-positive phenotype (indicating a reverse mutation in the histidine locus) is established by counting colonies that have been grown in histidine-free media. Inclusion of an exogenous metabolizing system (Aroclor induced rat liver S9 microsomal fraction) allows for the detection of mutagens requiring metabolic activation to form DNA-reactive intermediates. In addition to several strains of *S. typhimurium* (e.g.TA98, TA100, TA102, TA1535, TA1537, TA1538), each allowing detection of different mutation types, this assay has been adapted in a strain of *Escherichia coli* (WP2*uvr*A) to identify base-pair substitutions based on reversion at the tryptophan locus. Given the possible differences in cellular uptake of particulates and genomic complexity between prokaryotes and eukaryotes, genotoxicity data for nanomaterials obtained from the Ames assay should be interpreted carefully. The Ames assay should not be considered as a stand alone assay for identifying genotoxicity elicited by nanomaterials in humans and other vertebrates, and should instead be supplemented with additional studies as described hereafter.

2.2. Cytogenetic Assessment of Chromosome Damage through Analysis of Chromosomal Aberration Induction and Micronuclei

In addition to determining mutations of a particular gene, it is important to evaluate effects on the number and integrity of chromosomes via karyotype analyses. Such analyses can be carried out directly via simple staining techniques (5% Giemsa) and microscopy, and entail evaluation of changes in the morphological appearance of chromosomes (chromosomal aberrations representing clastogenicity) and the presence of micronuclei. Protocols typically involve treatment of cells during S-phase (due to the sensitivity of cells at this point in the cell cycle) followed by treatment at predetermined intervals with a substance such as Colcemid® or colchicine that is capable of arresting the cells in metaphase. Alternatively, assessment of chromosomal breakage and chromosome loss events can be carried out by identifying the presence of micronuclei. Micronuclei are chromosomal fragments or whole chromosomes that are not incorporated into the nucleus of either daughter cell at anaphase, and are therefore bound by a membrane and remain in the cytoplasm through subsequent cell cycles. Micronucleus assays typically employ a cytokinesis-block technique in which cytochalasin B is used to inhibit cytokinesis, thus allowing micronuclei to be assessed in binucleated cells. This is important since micronuclei are most accurately quantified in bi nucleated cells that have undergone only one cell division. Karyotypic analyses as described above have been carried out for a number of nanomaterials.

2.3. Comet Assay

The single cell gel electrophoresis (comet) assay is technically simple, relatively fast, cheap, and DNA damage can be investigated in virtually all mammalian cell types without requirement for cell culture. The comet assay can be employed as a genotoxicity test in evaluating the genetic toxicology of environmental agents, encompassing both experimental animal models and biomonitoring. The simple version of the alkaline comet assay detects DNA migration caused by strand breaks, alkaline labile sites, and transient repair sites. The pH > 13 version is capable of detecting DNA single-strand breaks (SSB), alkali-labile sites (ALS), DNA-DNA/DNA-protein cross-linking, and SSB associated with incomplete excision repair sites. Relative to other genotoxicity tests, the advantages of the SCG assay include its demonstrated sensitivity for detecting low levels of DNA damage, requirement for small numbers of cells per sample, its flexibility, its low costs, its ease of application, and the short time needed to complete a study. The cells are embedded in agarose and lysed, generating nucleus-like structures in the gel (referred to as nucleoids). Following alkaline electrophoresis, the DNA strands migrate toward the anode, and the extent of migration depends on the number of SB in the nucleoids. The migration is visualized and scored in a fluorescence microscope after staining.

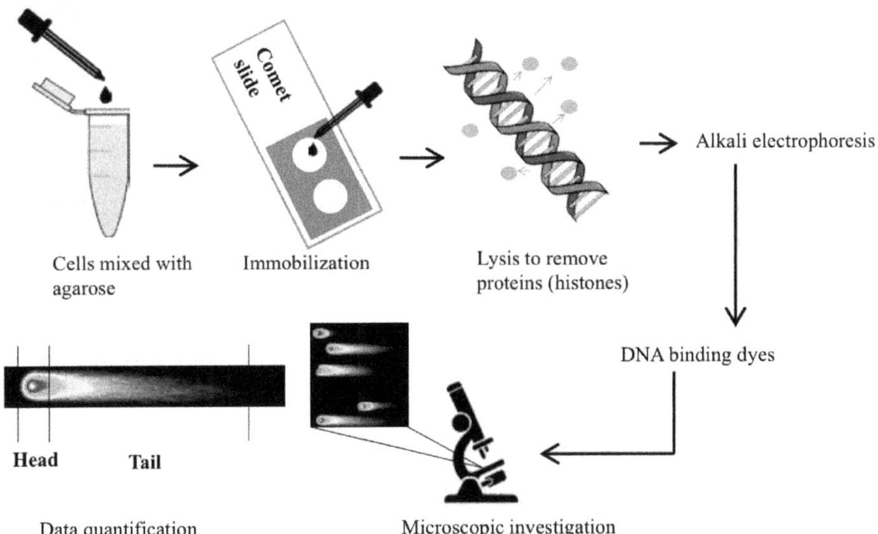

2.4. 8-Oxo-dG Assay

Oxidative damage in DNA has often been suggested as a contributing factor in the process of aging and the development of cancer. One of the most studied and important lesions produced in DNA by reactive oxygen species is 7-hydro-8-oxodeoxyguanosine (8-oxodG). Due to its mispairing with deoxyadenosine, 8-oxodG is mutagenic. Also, 8-OxodG was found to be highly miscoding during replication with purified DNA polymerases *in vitro*. 8-oxodG is not poorly repaired in the cells, causing a block of DNA replication. The production of 8-Hydroxyguanine (8-oxo-dG) is almost exclusively elicited by oxidative stress. Polymerases preferentially insert adenine opposite 8-oxo-dG. Therefore, oxidatively damaged adducts, without repair, are susceptible to G to T transitions.

In *Escherichia coli*, 8-oxodG is removed from DNA by either a specific glycosylase, known as formamidopyrimidine glycosylase (Fpg protein), in the initial step of base excision repair (BER), or by the UvrABC enzymes through nucleotide excision repair (NER). Cells deficient in either pathway do not show an appreciable defect in the repair of 8-oxodG, but the double mutants exhibit sensitivity to agents producing 8oxodG lesions. Eukaryotic cells may also employ multiple pathways for the removal of this common lesion. When the cells fail to remove the lesion it leads to misincorporation, mutagenicity and genotoxicity.

2.5. Quantification of 8- Oxo-dG

8-hydroxy-2-deoxy Guanosine (8-OH-dG) is a product of oxidative damage of DNA by reactive oxygen and nitrogen species and serves as an established marker of oxidative stress. Hydroxylation of guanosine occurs in response to both normal metabolic processes and a variety of environmental factors. Increased levels of 8-OH-dG are associated with the aging process as well as with a number of pathological conditions including cancer, diabetes, and hypertension. 8-OH-dG can be quantified in EIA which is a competitive assay which can be performed in cell culture, plasma, microbial lysates and other sample matrices. The EIA utilizes an anti-mouse IgG-coated plate and a tracer consisting of an 8-OH-dG-enzyme conjugate. This format has the advantage of providing low variability and increased sensitivity compared to assays that utilize an antigen-coated plate.

3. Assays for Alteration in Gene Expression

Gene expression assays, i.e., gene profiling, are an important tool for screening different environmental particles, including nanoparticles. Techniques used to assess gene expression include: Northern blot analysis, quantitative real-time polymerase chain reaction (qRT-PCR), PCR arrays and micro arrays.

3.1. Real Time Polymerase Chain Reaction (RT-PCR)

Real-time PCR is a quantitative method for the determination of copy number of PCR templates, such as DNA or cDNA and consists of two types: probe-based and intercalator based. Probe-based real-time PCR, also known as Taqman PCR, requires a pair of PCR primers (as regular PCR does), and an additional fluorogenic oligonucleotide probe with both a reporter fluorescent dye and a quencher dye attached. The intercalator-based (SYBR Green) method requires a double-stranded DNA dye in the PCR reaction which binds to newly synthesized double-stranded DNA and renders fluorescence. Both methods require a special thermocycler equipped with a sensitive camera that monitors the fluorescence in each well of a 96-well plate at frequent intervals during the PCR reaction.

PCR arrays are important tools for analyzing the expression of a focused panel of genes. Each 96-well plate includes SYBR Green-optimized primer assays for a thoroughly researched panel of relevant, pathway-or disease-focused genes. In PCR arrays, 96 different gene-specific products are simultaneously amplified under uniform cycling conditions using specific master mix formulation and subsequently detected.

3.2. Micro array Analyses

Gene expression profiling by micro array analysis has enabled the measurement of mRNA levels of thousands of genes in a single RNA sample. In this technique, a glass slide or membrane is spotted or "arrayed" with DNA fragments or oligo nucleotides that represent specific gene coding regions. Purified RNA is then fluorescently or radioactively labeled and hybridized to the slide/membrane. After thorough washing, the raw data is obtained by laser scanning or auto radiographic imaging and subsequently entered into a database and analyzed by a number of statistical methods.

Closing Notes

Biosafety is integral to modern biotechnology. The adoption of modern biotech products needs to be balanced with adequate biosafety safeguards. Scientific risk assessment and cost benefit analysis have to be done by case by case studies individually. Biosafety panel of tests, need based adoption in NP products is recommended. Also the participation of scientists from various fields is important. Dissemination of knowledge and information occupy the integral part of Biosafety.

Self-assessment Questions

1. What is nano-toxicity ?
2. Narrate widely used assay for cytotoxicity
3. Define "Geno-toxicity"
4. Which is the model organism for "aquatic pollution"?
5. What are all the human cell lines used for assessing nano-toxicity
6. Importance of "Hydroxyguanine (8-oxo-dG)"
7. What is LD50?
8. Explain "Oxidative Stress"
9. Routes of NPs entry into humans
10. Expand OECD

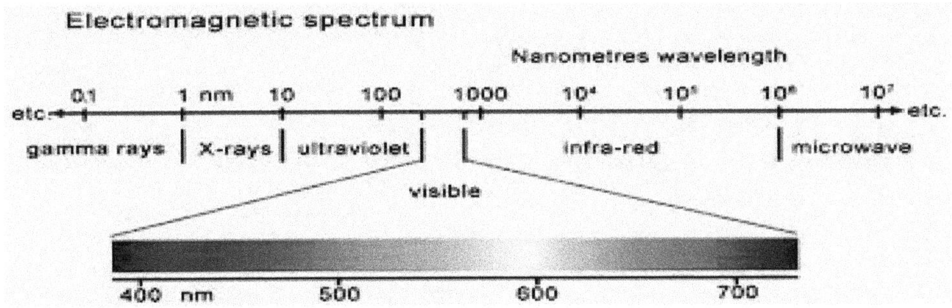

Fig. 1: Electromagnetic spectra in terms of wavelength (λ) (P. 103)

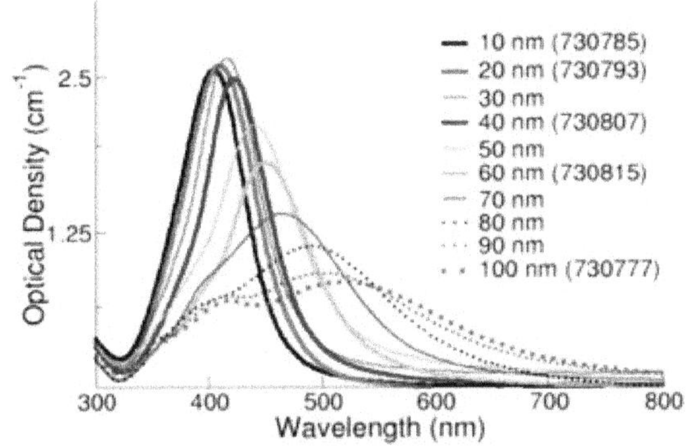

Fig. 4: Representation of UV spectra of silver nanoparticles at different concentration by observing wavelength (nm) in X-axis and Optical density (Cm^{-1}) in Y-axis. (P. 105)

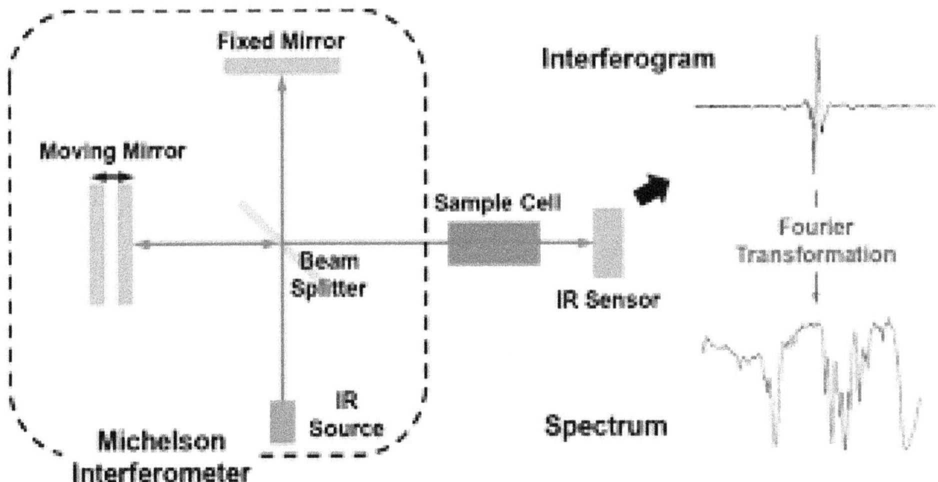

Fig. 1: Schematic representation of an Interferometer (P. 110)

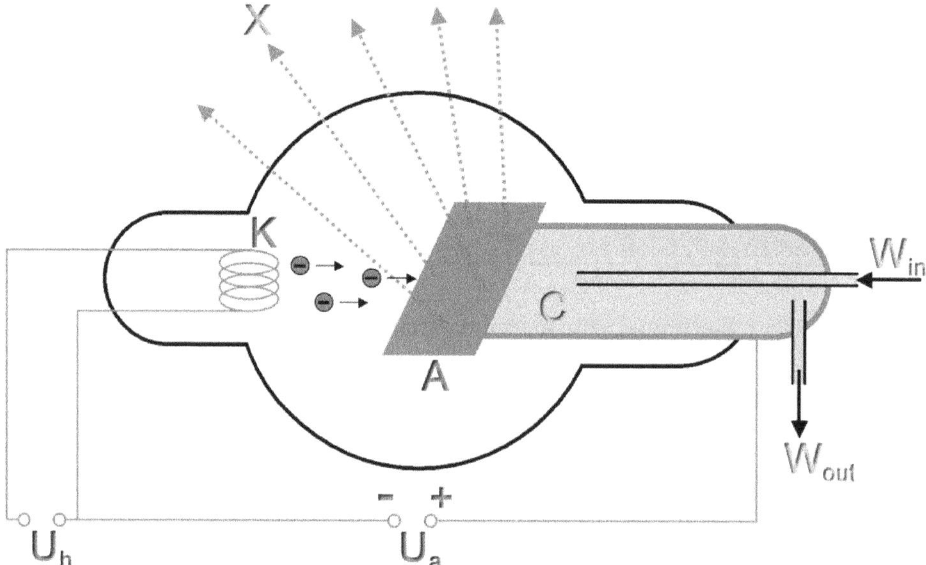

Fig.1:X-raytubeconsistsofK(cathode)andA(anodemostlymetaltargets)biasedwithpositive potential. C refers to chiller unit for dissipating heat from anodes and X are X- rays (P. 114)

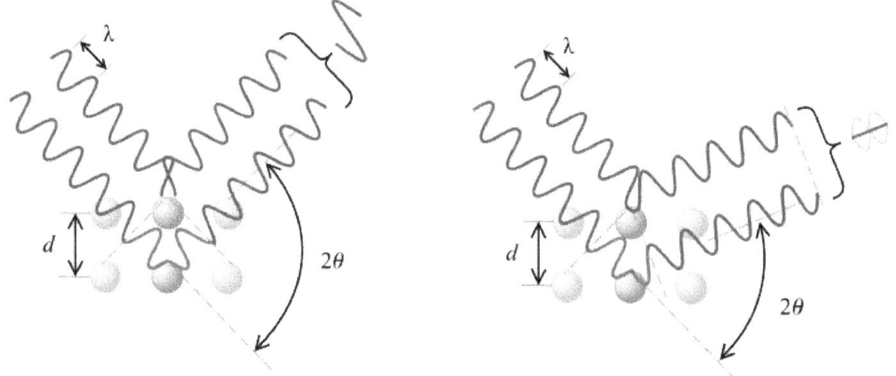

Fig 3: Constructive Interference (left) takes place when diffracted waves are in phase and destructive interference takes place (right) when diffracted waves are out of phase (P. 116)

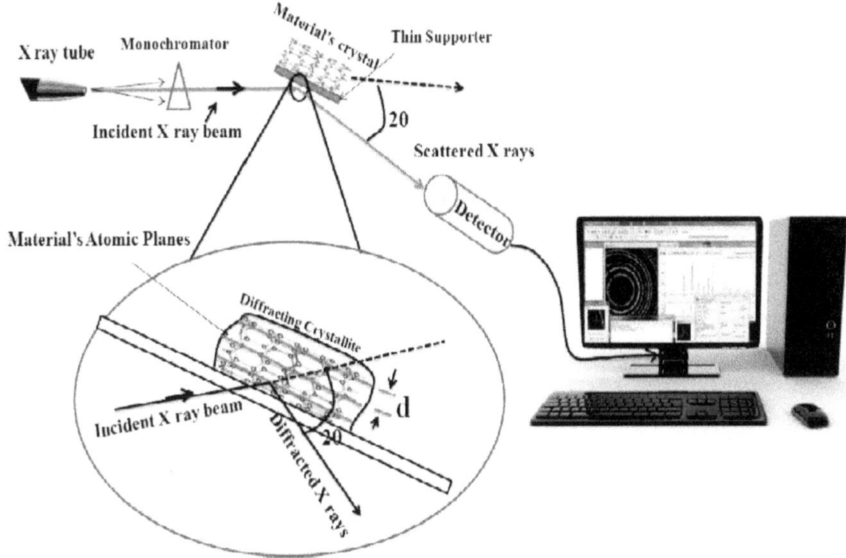

Fig. 6: Schematic illustration of X-ray Diffractometer (Adopted from Das *et al.,* 2014) (P. 120)

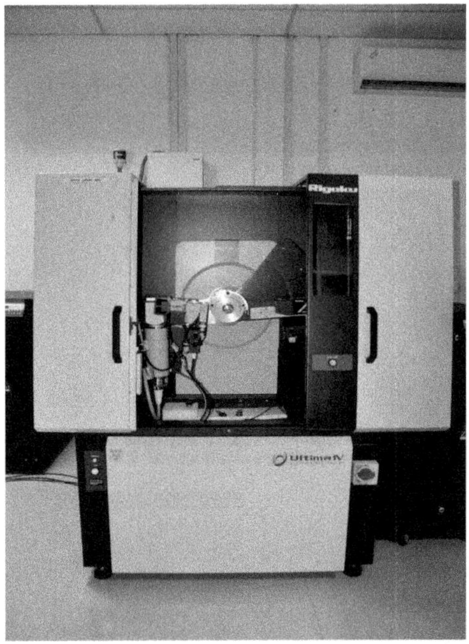

Fig. 7: X-ray Diffractometer (Rigaku Model Ultima IV) (P. 120)

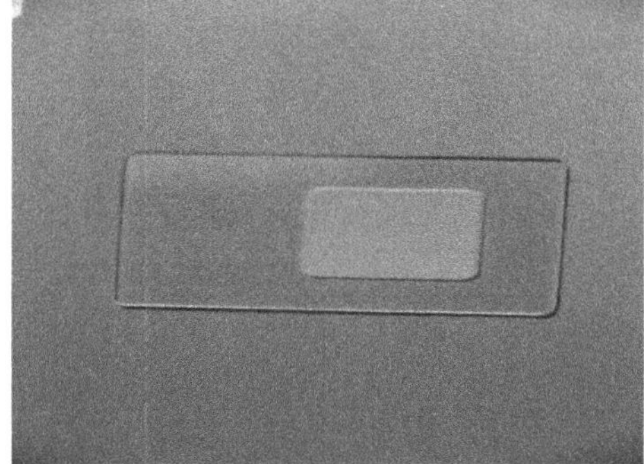

Fig. 8: Glass plate sample holder with designated area (depression) for filling sample (P. 121)

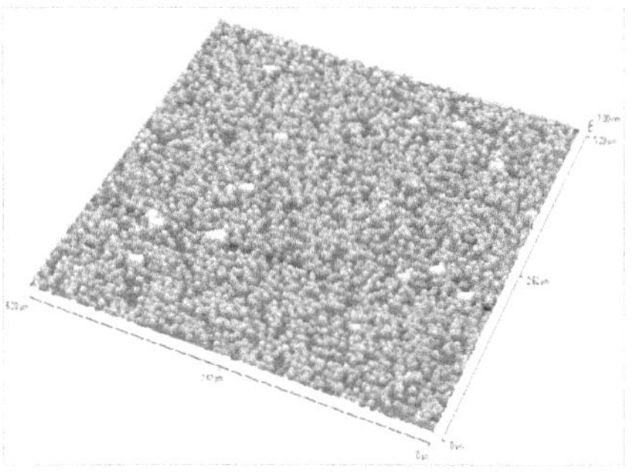
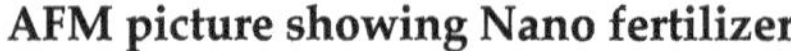

AFM picture showing Nano fertilizer

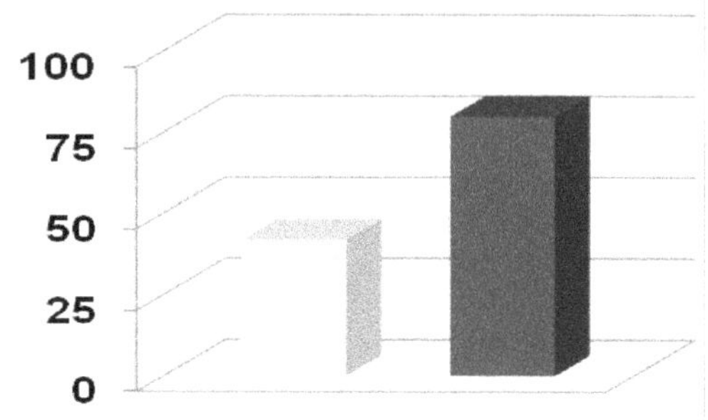

Relative performance of Nano-fertilizer

(P. 141)

Fig. 12. SEM images of Root Nodule

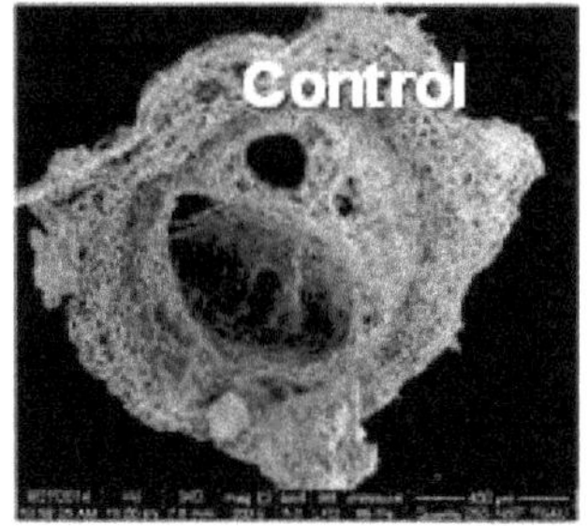

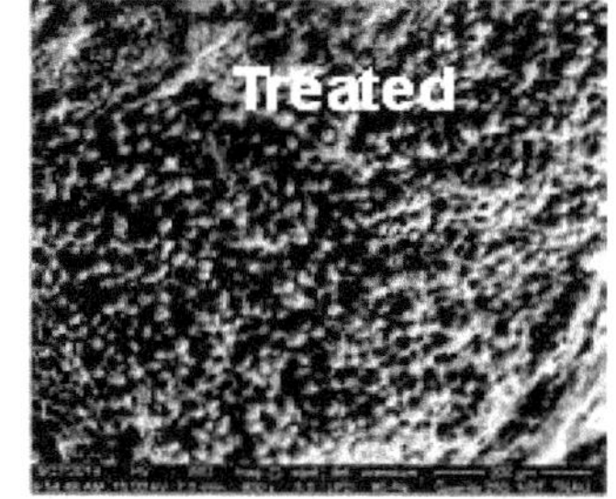

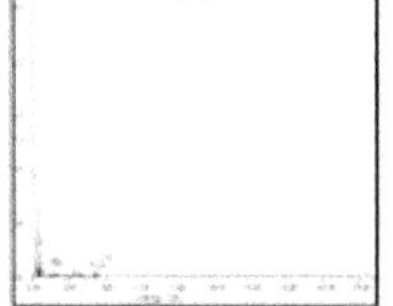

Element	Wt %	At %
C K	50.57	58.56
N K	10.26	10.11
O K	33.96	29.30
MgK	01.28	00.73
SK	0.83	0.36
K K	02.13	00.75
CaK	00.57	00.20

Element	Wt %	At %
N K	10.81	13.97
O K	64.57	73.09
MgK	02.41	01.80
AlK	03.16	02.12
SK	2.43	1.37
K K	11.92	05.52
CaK	04.71	02.13

Root Nodules of Nano-S fertilized Groundnut Plants (P. 144)

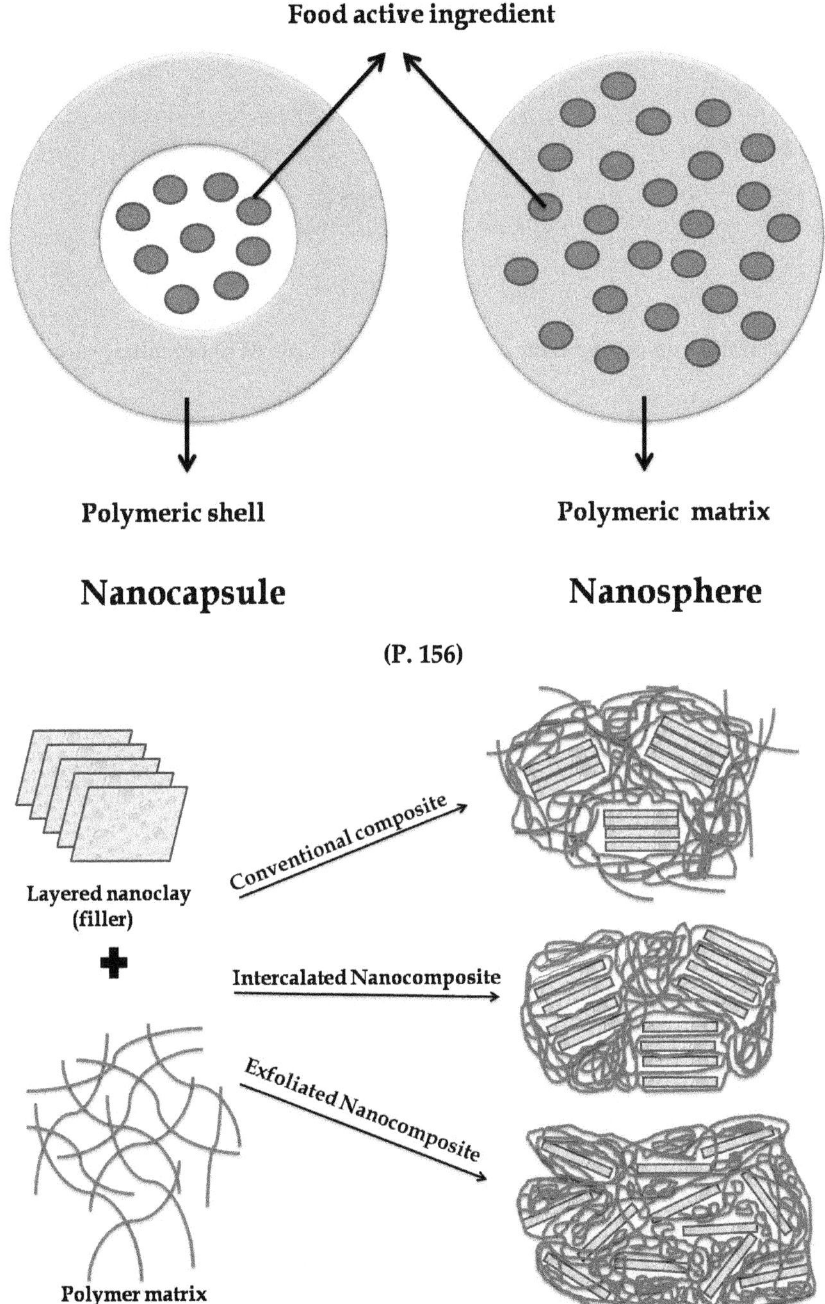

(P. 156)

Fig. 2: Graphical representation on types of nanocomposites formed from polymer matrix and layered nanoclay (Credit: Haripriya Shanmugam and Preetha Sundharam)

(P. 160)

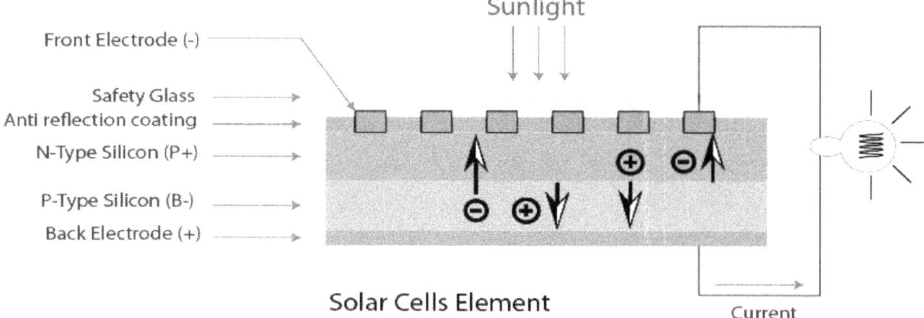

Fig. 2: Illustration on components and working principle of photovoltaic cells (P. 164)

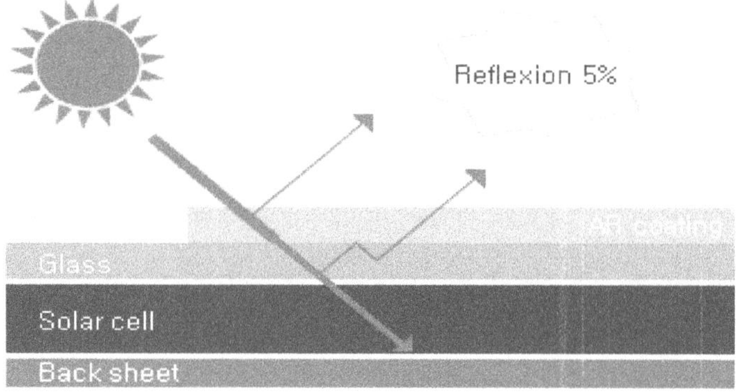

Fig. 2: AR refers to antireflective coating which improve transmission of light reducing refection from the surface (P. 165)

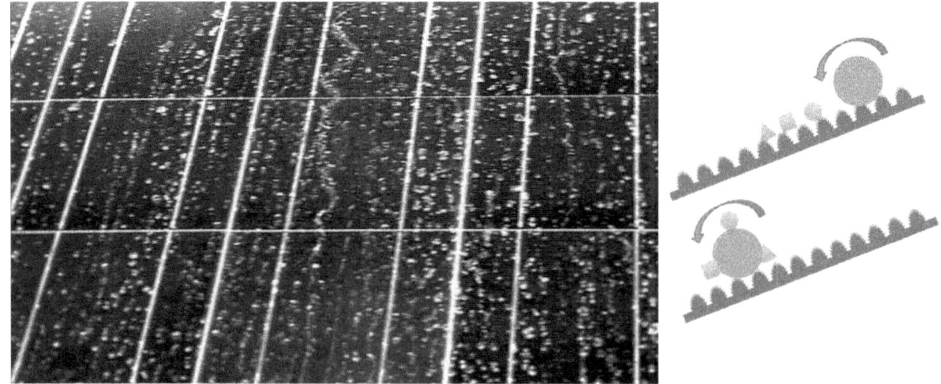

Fig. 3: Self-cleaning solar panels for dust free in panels (Courtesy: University of Houston) and mechanism of self-cleaning *(Courtesy: He, 2016, P.No 9)* (P. 166)

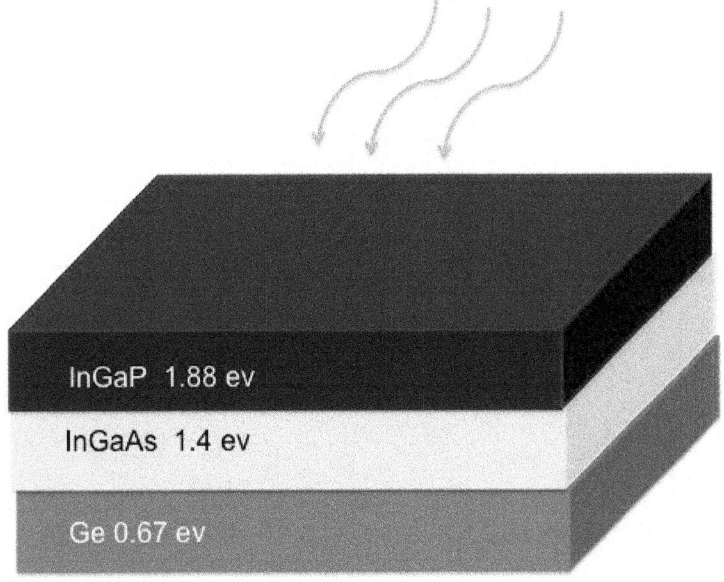

Fig. 4: Tandem solar cells of multiple materials with different band gaps (P. 166)

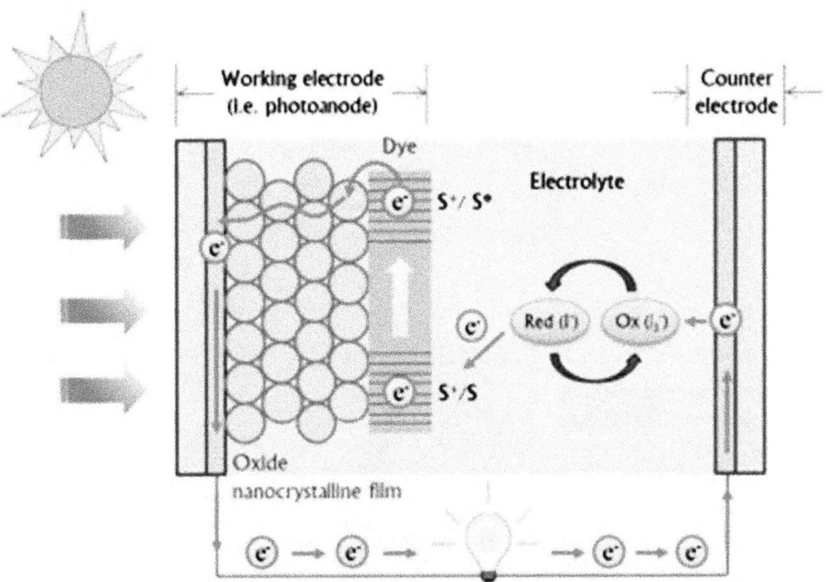

Fig. 5: Illustration on the working of dye sensitized solar cells (P. 167)

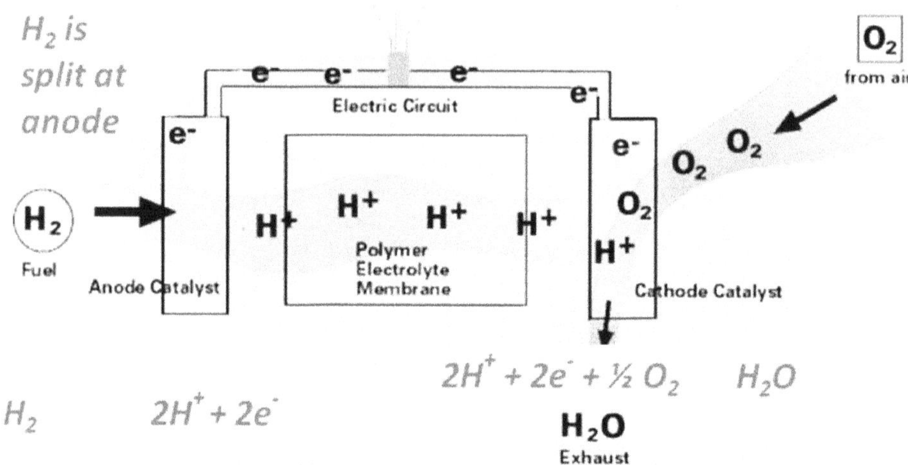

Fig 6: Fuel cells consists of cathode and anode separated with polymer electrolyte membrane where hydrogen is split at anode through electro oxidation releasing electrons and protons reaching cathode where both combines with oxygen to form water (P. 169)

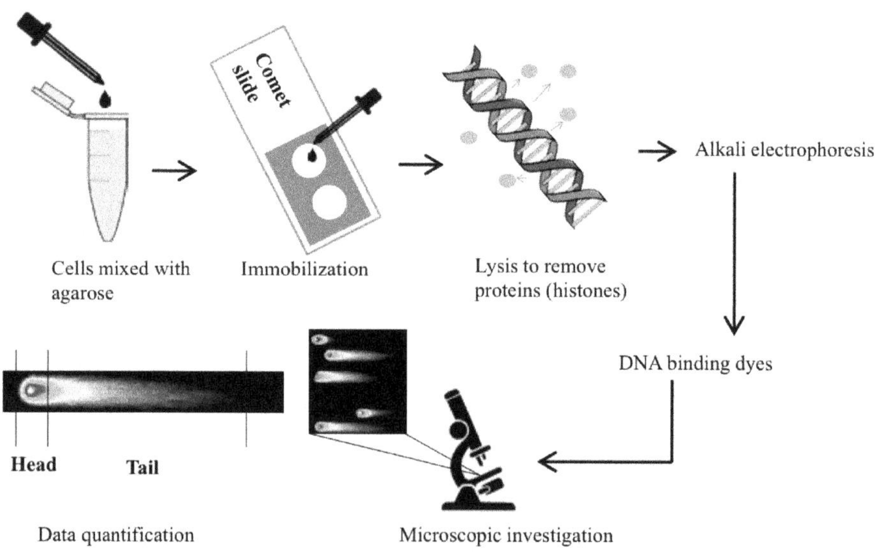

(P. 185)

www.ingramcontent.com/pod-product-compliance
Ingram Content Group UK Ltd.
Pitfield, Milton Keynes, MK11 3LW, UK
UKHW021948270726
14060UKWH00002B/415

9 789390 384600